RENAL DIET COOKBOOK:

200+ Delicious Recipes, Easy And Quick To Prepare For Those Who Have Dialysis & 21-Day Meal Plan.

TABLE OF CONTENTS

Introduction

Human health hangs in a complete balance when all of its interconnected bodily mechanisms function properly in perfect sync. Without its major organs working normally, the body soon suffers indelible damage. Kidney malfunction is one such example, and it is not just the entire water balance that is disturbed by the kidney disease, but a number of other diseases also emerge due to this problem. Kidney diseases are progressive in nature, meaning that if left unchecked and uncontrolled, they can ultimately lead to permanent kidney damage. That is why it is essential to control and manage the disease and put a halt to its progress, which can be done through medicinal and natural means. While medicines can guarantee only thirty percent of the cure, a change of lifestyle and diet can prove to be miraculous with their seventy percent of guaranteed results. A kidney-friendly diet and lifestyle not only saves the kidneys from excess minerals, but it also aids medicines to work actively. Treatment without a good diet, hence, proves to be useless. In this renal diet cookbook, we shall bring out the basic facts about kidney diseases, their symptoms, causes, and diagnosis. This preliminary introduction can help the readers understand the problem clearly; then, we shall discuss the role of renal diet and kidney-friendly lifestyle in curbing the diseases. And it's not just that, the book also contains a range of delicious renal diet recipes which will guarantee luscious flavors and good health.

Despite their tiny size, the kidneys perform a number of functions which are vital for the body to be able to function healthily.

These include:

- Filtering excess fluids and waste from the blood
- Creating the enzyme known as renin which regulates blood pressure,
- Ensuring bone marrow creates red blood cells,
- Controlling calcium and phosphorus levels through absorption and excretion.

Unfortunately, when kidney disease reaches a chronic stage, these functions start to stop working. However, with the right treatment and lifestyle, it is possible to manage symptoms and continue living well. This is even more applicable in the earlier stages of the disease. Tactlessly, 10% of all adults over the age of 20 will experience some form of kidney disease in their lifetime. There are a variety of different treatments for kidney disease, which depend on the cause of the disease.

Kidney (or renal) diseases are affecting around 14% of the adult population according to international stats. In the US, approx. 661.000 Americans suffer from kidney dysfunction. Out of these patients, 468.000 proceed to dialysis treatment and the rest have one active kidney transplant.

The high quantities of diabetes and heart illness are additionally related with kidney dysfunction and sometimes one condition for example diabetes may prompt the other.

With such a significant number of high rates, possibly the best course of treatment is the contravention of dialysis, which makes people depend upon clinical and crisis facility meds in any occasion multiple times every week. In this manner, if your kidney has just given a few indications of brokenness, you can forestall dialysis through eating routine, something that we will talk about in this book.

CHAPTER 1:

Chronic Kidney Disease

Kidneys are important organs for the human body. They filter out excess water, waste products, and other impurities of the blood. Chronic kidney disease or CKD means your kidneys are damaged and can't filter blood properly. The kidney damage can cause waste to build up in your body. CKD causes many health problem.

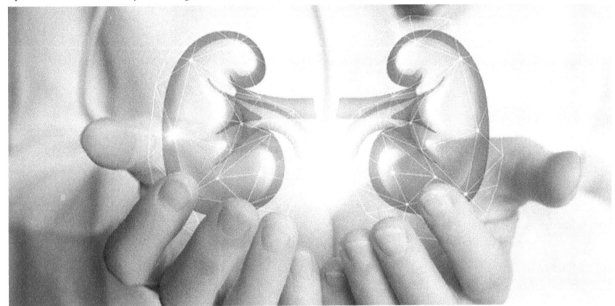

Who is at risk of developing CKD?

1. Diabetes: People with diabetes are prone to CKD. Data shows that about one-third of diabetic patients have CKD.

2. High blood pressure: About 1 in 5 adults with high blood pressure has CKD.

3. Heart disease: Recent research shows that there is a link between high blood pressure and kidney disease. People with kidney disease are at a higher risk of heart disease and people with heart disease are at a higher risk of kidney disease.

4. Family history of kidney failure: People with a family history are at risk for CKD.

Besides this there are other risk factors including

*   Being Asian-American, Native American, And African-American

*   Smoking

*   Old age

*   Obesity

Symptoms of CKD

Early stages of chronic kidney disease may not have any symptoms. It is because even if your kidney is damaged, it can still do enough work to keep you healthy. The blood and urine tests are the only ways to know if you have kidney disease.

 Symptoms of advanced CKD

- Weight loss
- Vomiting
- Trouble concentrating
- Sleep problems
- Shortness of breath
- Nausea
- Muscle cramps
- Loss of appetite
- Increased or decreased urination
- Headaches
- Feeling tired
- Itching or numbness
- Dry skin
- Chest pain

A brief snapshot of each stage:

Stage 1: Considered the normal or high risk of developing CKD. The Glomerular Filtration Rate (GFR) falls > 90 mL/min.

Stage 2: Considered as mild CKD. The GFR falls in the range of 60-89 mL/min.

Stage 3: Moderate CKD which ranges from 45-59 mL/min.

Stage 4: Severe Chronic Kidney disease. Rates fall between 15-29 mL/min.

Stage 5: Final/end-stage of the renal disease which calls for surgery or dialysis. Also called End Stage Renal Disease (ESRD). The GFR levels, in this case, fall below 15 mL/min.

Causes of Kidney Disease?

There are many causes of kidney disease, including physical injury or disorders that can damage the kidneys, but the two leading causes of kidney disease are diabetes and high blood pressure. These underlying conditions also put people at risk for developing cardiovascular disease. Early treatment may not only slow down the progression of the disease, but also reduce your risk of developing heart disease or stroke.

Kidney disease can affect anyone, at any age. African Americans, Hispanics, and American Indians are at increased risk for kidney failure, because these groups have a greater prevalence of diabetes and high blood pressure.

Uncontrolled diabetes is the leading cause of kidney disease. Diabetes can damage the kidneys and cause them to fail.

The second leading cause of kidney disease is high blood pressure, also known as hypertension. One in three Americans is at risk for kidney disease because of hypertension. Although there is no cure for hypertension, certain medications, a low-sodium diet, and physical activity can lower blood pressure.

The kidneys help manage blood pressure, but when blood pressure is high, the heart has to work overtime at pumping blood. When the force of blood flow is high, blood vessels start to stretch so the blood can flow more easily. The stretching and scarring weakens the blood vessels throughout the entire body, including the kidneys. And when the kidneys' blood vessels are injured, they may not remove the waste and extra fluid from the body, creating a dangerous cycle, because the extra fluid in the blood vessels can increase blood pressure even more.

Cardiovascular disease is the leading cause of death in the United States. When kidney disease occurs, that process can be affected, and the risk of developing heart disease becomes greater. Cardiovascular disease is an umbrella term used to describe conditions that may damage the heart and blood vessels, including coronary artery disease, heart attack, heart failure, atherosclerosis, and high blood pressure. Complications from renal disease may develop, and can lead to heart disease.

With diabetes, excess blood sugar remains in the bloodstream. The high blood sugar levels can damage the blood vessels in the kidneys and elsewhere in the body. And since high blood pressure is a complication from diabetes, the extra pressure can weaken the walls of the blood vessels, which can lead to a heart attack or stroke.

Other conditions, such as drug abuse and certain autoimmune diseases, can also cause injury to the kidneys. In fact, every drug we put into our body has to pass through the kidneys for filtration. If the drug is not taken following a healthcare provider's instructions, or if it is an illegal substance such as heroin, cocaine, or ecstasy, it can cause injury to the kidneys by raising the blood pressure, also increasing the risk of a stroke, heart failure, and even death.

An autoimmune disease is one in which the immune system, designed to protect the body from illness, sees the body as an invader and attacks its own systems, including the kidneys. Some forms of lupus, for example, attack the kidneys. Another autoimmune disease that can lead to kidney failure is Good pasture syndrome, a group of conditions that affect the kidneys and the lungs. The damage to the kidneys from autoimmune diseases can lead to chronic kidney disease and kidney failure.

Diagnosis tests

Besides identifying the symptoms of kidney disease, there are other better and more accurate ways to confirm the extent of loss of renal function. There are mainly two important diagnostic tests:

1. Urine test

The urine test clearly states all the renal problems. The urine is the waste product of the kidney. When there is loss of filtration or any hindrance to the kidneys, the urine sample will indicate it through the number of excretory products present in it. The severe stages of chronic disease show some amount of protein and blood in the urine. Do not rely on self-tests; visit an authentic clinic for these tests.

2. Blood pressure and blood test

Another good way to check for renal disease is to test the blood and its composition. A high amount of creatinine and other waste products in the blood clearly indicates that the kidneys are not functioning properly. Blood pressure can also be indicative of renal disease. When the water balance in the body is disturbed, it may cause high blood pressure. Hypertension can both be the cause and symptom of kidney disease and therefore should be taken seriously.

Treatment

The best way to manage CKD is to be an active participant in your treatment program, regardless of your stage of renal disease. Proper treatment involves a combination of working with a healthcare team, adhering to a renal diet, and making healthy lifestyle decisions. These can all have a profoundly positive effect on your kidney disease—especially watching how you eat.

Working with your healthcare team. When you have kidney disease, working in partnership with your healthcare team can be extremely important in your treatment program as well as being personally empowering. Regularly meeting with your physician or healthcare team can arm you with resources and information that help you make informed decisions regarding your treatment needs, and provide you with a much needed opportunity to vent, share information, get advice, and receive support in effectively managing this illness.

Adhering to a renal diet. The heart of this book is the renal diet. Sticking to this diet can make a huge difference in your health and vitality. Like any change, following the diet may not be easy at first. Important changes to your diet, particularly early on, can possibly prevent the need for dialysis. These changes include limiting salt, eating a low-protein diet, reducing fat intake, and getting enough calories if you need to lose weight. Be honest with yourself first and foremost—learn what you need, and consider your personal goals and obstacles. Start by making small changes. It is okay to have some slip-ups—we all do. With guidance and support, these small changes will become habits of your promising new lifestyle. In no time, you will begin taking control of your diet and health.

Making healthy lifestyle decisions. Lifestyle choices play a crucial part in our health, especially when it comes to helping regulate kidney disease. Lifestyle choices such as allotting time for physical activity, getting enough sleep, managing weight, reducing stress, and limiting smoking and alcohol will help you take control of your overall health, making it easier to manage your kidney disease. Follow this simple formula: Keep toxins out of your body as much as you can, and build up your immune system with a good balance of exercise, relaxation, and sleep.

CHAPTER 2:

Recommended Foods

There are many foods that work well within the renal diet, and once you see the available variety, it will not seem as restrictive or difficult to follow. The key is focusing on the foods with a high level of nutrients, which make it easier for the kidneys to process waste by not adding too much that the body needs to discard. Balance is a major factor in maintaining and improving long-term renal function.

Garlic

An excellent, vitamin-rich food for the immune system, garlic is a tasty substitute for salt in a variety of dishes. It acts as a significant source of vitamin C and B6, while aiding the kidneys in ridding the body of unwanted toxins. It's a great, healthy way to add flavor for skillet meals, pasta, soups, and stews.

Berries

All berries are considered a good renal diet food due to their high level of fiber, antioxidants, and delicious taste, making them an easy option to include as a light snack or as an ingredient in smoothies, salads, and light desserts. Just one handful of blueberries can provide almost one day's vitamin C requirement, as well as a boost of fiber, which is good for weight loss and maintenance.

Bell Peppers

Flavorful and easy to enjoy both raw and cooked, bell peppers offer a good source of vitamin C, vitamin A, and fiber. Along with other kidney-friendly foods, they make the detoxification process much easier while boosting your body's nutrient level to prevent further health conditions and reduce existing deficiencies.

Onions

This nutritious and tasty vegetable is excellent as a companion to garlic in many dishes, or on its own. Like garlic, onions can provide flavor as an alternative to salt, and provides a good source of vitamin C, vitamin B, manganese, and fiber, as well. Adding just one quarter or half of an onion is often enough for most meals, because of its strong, pungent flavor.

Macadamia Nuts

If you enjoy nuts and seeds as snacks, you many soon learn that many contain high amounts of phosphorus and should be avoided or limited as much as possible. Fortunately, macadamia nuts are an easier option to digest and process, as they contain much lower amounts of phosphorus and make an excellent substitute for other nuts. They are a good source of other nutrients, as well, such as vitamin B, copper, manganese, iron, and healthy fats.

Pineapple

Unlike other fruits that are high in potassium, pineapple is an option that can be enjoyed more often than bananas and kiwis. Citrus fruits are generally high in potassium. If you find yourself craving an orange or grapefruit, choose pineapple instead. In addition to providing a high levels of vitamin B and fiber, pineapples can reduce inflammation thanks to an enzyme called brome lain.

Mushrooms

In general, mushrooms are a safe, healthy option for the renal diet, especially the shiitake variety, high in nutrients such as selenium, vitamin B, and manganese. They contain a moderate amount of plant-based protein, which is easier for your body to digest and use than animal proteins. Shiitake and Portobello mushrooms are often used in vegan diets as a meat substitute, due to their texture and pleasant flavor.

CHAPTER 3:

Foods to Avoid

Eating restrictions might be different depending upon your level of kidney disease. If you are in the early stages of kidney disease, you may have different restrictions as compared to those who are at the end-stage renal disease, or kidney failure. In contrast to this, people with an end-stage renal disease requiring dialysis will face different eating restrictions. Let's discuss some of the foods to avoid while being on the renal diet.

Dark-Colored Colas contain calories, sugar, phosphorus, etc. They contain phosphorus to enhance flavor, increase its life and avoid discoloration. Which can be found in a product's ingredient list. This addition of phosphorus varies depending on the type of cola. Mostly, the dark-colored colas contain 50–100 mg in a 200-ml serving. Therefore, dark colas should be avoided on a renal diet.

Canned Foods including soups, vegetables, and beans, are low in cost but contain high amounts of sodium due to the addition of salt to increase its life. Due to this amount of sodium inclusion in canned goods, people with kidney disease should avoid consumption. Opt for lower-sodium content with the label "no salt added". One more way is to drain or rinse canned foods, such as canned beans and tuna, could decrease the sodium content by 33–80%, depending on the product.

One cup already cooked brown rice possesses about 150 mg of phosphorus and 154 mg of potassium, whereas, one cup of already cooked white rice has about 69 mg of phosphorus and 54 mg of potassium. Bulgur, buckwheat, pearled barley and couscous are equally beneficial, low-phosphorus options and might be a good alternative instead of brown rice.

Bananas are high potassium content, low in sodium, and provides 422 mg of potassium per banana. It might disturb your daily balanced potassium intake to 2,000 mg if a banana is a daily staple.

Whole-Wheat Bread may harm individuals with kidney disease. But for healthy individuals, it is recommended over refined, white flour bread. White bread is recommended instead of whole-wheat varieties for individuals with kidney disease because it has phosphorus and potassium. If you add more bran and whole grains in the bread, then the amount of phosphorus and potassium contents increases.

Oranges and Orange Juice are enriched with vitamin C content and potassium. 184 grams provides 333 mg of potassium and 473 mg of potassium in one cup of orange juice. With these calculations, oranges and orange juice must be avoided or used in a limited amount while being on a renal diet.

If you are suffering from or living with kidney disease, reducing your potassium, phosphorus and sodium intake is an essential aspect of managing and tackling the disease. The foods with high-potassium, high-sodium, and high-phosphorus content listed above should always be limited or avoided. These restrictions and nutrients intakes may differ depending on the level of damage to your kidneys. Following a renal diet might be a daunting procedure and a restrictive one most of the times. But, working with your physician and nutrition specialist and a renal dietitian can assist you to formulate a renal diet specific to your individual needs.

CHAPTER 4:

Breakfast

1. Garlic Mayo Bread

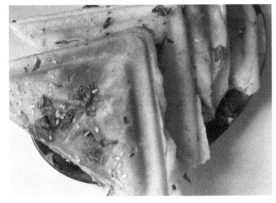

Preparation Time: 10 minutes

Cooking Time: 5 minutes

Servings: 16

Ingredients:

- 3 tablespoons vegetable oil
- 4 cloves garlic, minced
- 2 teaspoons paprika
- Dash cayenne pepper
- 1 teaspoon lemon juice
- 2 tablespoons Parmesan cheese, grated
- 3/4 cup mayonnaise
- 1 loaf (1 lb.) French bread, sliced
- 1 teaspoon Italian herbs

Directions:

1. Mix the garlic with the oil in a small bowl and leave it overnight.
2. Discard the garlic from the bowl and keep the garlic-infused oil.
3. Mix the garlic-oil with cayenne, paprika, lemon juice, mayonnaise, and Parmesan.
4. Place the bread slices in a baking tray lined with parchment paper.
5. Top these slices with the mayonnaise mixture and drizzle the Italian herbs on top.
6. Broil these slices for 5 minutes until golden brown.
7. Serve warm.

Nutrition:

Calories 217, Total Fat 7.9g,

Sodium 423mg, Dietary Fiber 1.3g,

Sugars 2g, Protein 7g, Calcium 56mg,

Phosphorous 347mg, Potassium 72mg

2. Strawberry Topped Waffles

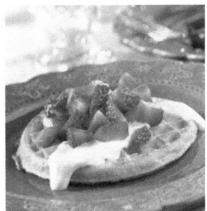

Preparation Time: 15 minutes

Cooking Time: 20 minutes

Servings: 5

Ingredients:

- 1 cup flour
- 1/4 cup Swerve

- 1 ¾ teaspoons baking powder
- 1 egg, separated
- ¾ cup milk
- ½ cup butter, melted
- ½ teaspoon vanilla extract
- Fresh strawberries, sliced

Directions:

1. Prepare and preheat your waffle pan following the instructions of the machine.
2. Begin by mixing the flour with Swerve and baking soda in a bowl.
3. Separate the egg yolks from the egg whites, keeping them in two separate bowls.
4. Add the milk and vanilla extract to the egg yolks.
5. Stir the melted butter and mix well until smooth.
6. Now beat the egg whites with an electric beater until foamy and fluffy.
7. Fold this fluffy composition in the egg yolk mixture.
8. Mix it gently until smooth, then add in the flour mixture.
9. Stir again to make a smooth mixture.
10. Pour a half cup of the waffle batter in a preheated pan and cook until the waffle is cooked.
11. Cook more waffles with the remaining batter.
12. Serve fresh with strawberries on top.

Nutrition:

Calories 342,

Total Fat 20.5g,

Sodium 156mg,

Dietary Fiber 0.7g,

Sugars 3.5g,

Protein 4.8g,

Calcium 107mg,

Phosphorous 126mg,

Potassium 233mg

3. Cheese Spaghetti Frittata

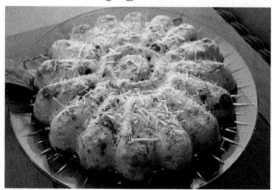

Preparation Time: 10 minutes

Cooking Time: 10 minutes

Servings: 6

Ingredients:

- 4 cups whole-wheat spaghetti, cooked
- 4 teaspoons olive oil
- 3 medium onions, chopped
- 4 large eggs
- 1/2 cup milk
- 1/3 cup Parmesan cheese, grated
- 2 tablespoons fresh parsley, chopped
- 2 tablespoons fresh basil, chopped
- 1/2 teaspoon black pepper
- 1 tomato, diced

Directions:

1. Set a suitable non-stick skillet over moderate heat and add in the olive oil.
2. Place the spaghetti in the skillet and cook by stirring for 2 minutes on moderate heat.
3. Whisk the eggs with milk, parsley, and black pepper in a bowl.

4. Pour this milky egg mixture over the spaghetti and top it all with basil, cheese, and tomato.

5. Cover the spaghetti frittata again with a lid and cook for approximately 8 minutes on low heat.

6. Slice and serve.

Nutrition:

Calories 230,

Total Fat 7.8g,

Sodium 77mg,

Dietary Fiber 5.6g,

Sugars 4.5g,

Protein 11.1g,

Calcium 88mg,

Phosphorous 368 mg,

Potassium 214mg,

4. Shrimp Bruschetta

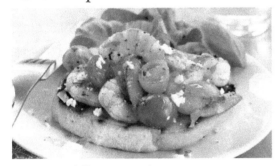

Preparation Time: 15 minutes

Cooking time: 10 minutes

Servings: 4

Ingredients:

- 13 oz. shrimps, peeled
- 1 tablespoon tomato sauce
- ½ teaspoon Splenda
- ¼ teaspoon garlic powder
- 1 teaspoon fresh parsley, chopped
- ½ teaspoon olive oil
- 1 teaspoon lemon juice

- 4 whole-grain bread slices
- 1 cup water, for cooking

Directions:

1. In the saucepan, pour water and bring it to boil.

2. Add shrimps and boil them over the high heat for 5 minutes.

3. After this, drain shrimps and chill them to the room temperature.

4. Mix up together shrimps with Splenda, garlic powder, tomato sauce, and fresh parsley.

5. Add lemon juice and stir gently.

6. Preheat the oven to 360f.

7. Coat the slice of bread with olive oil and bake for 3 minutes.

8. Then place the shrimp mixture on the bread. Bruschetta is cooked.

Nutrition:

Calories 199, Fat 3.7, Fiber 2.1,

Carbs 15.3, Protein 24.1

5. Strawberry Muesli

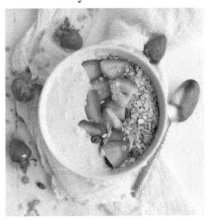

Preparation Time: 10 minutes

Cooking time: 30 minutes

Servings: 4

Ingredients:

- 2 cups Greek yogurt
- 1 ½ cup strawberries, sliced

- 1 ½ cup Muesli
- 4 teaspoon maple syrup
- ¾ teaspoon ground cinnamon

Directions:

1. Put Greek yogurt in the food processor.
2. Add 1 cup of strawberries, maple syrup, and ground cinnamon.
3. Blend the ingredients until you get smooth mass.
4. Transfer the yogurt mass in the serving bowls.
5. Add Muesli and stir well.
6. Leave the meal for 30 minutes in the fridge.
7. After this, decorate it with remaining sliced strawberries.

Nutrition:

Calories 149, Fat 2.6, Fiber 3.6,

Carbs 21.6, Protein 12

6. Yogurt Bulgur

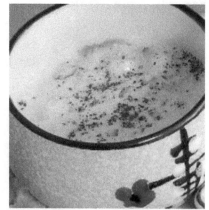

Preparation Time: 10 minutes

Cooking time: 15 minutes

Servings: 3

Ingredients:

- 1 cup bulgur
- 2 cups Greek yogurt

- 1 ½ cup water
- ½ teaspoon salt
- 1 teaspoon olive oil

Directions:

1. Pour olive oil in the saucepan and add bulgur.
2. Roast it over the medium heat for 2-3 minutes. Stir it from time to time.
3. After this, add salt and water.
4. Close the lid and cook bulgur for 15 minutes over the medium heat.
5. Then chill the cooked bulgur well and combine it with Greek yogurt. Stir it carefully.
6. Transfer the cooked meal into the serving plates. The yogurt bulgur tastes the best when it is cold.

Nutrition:

Calories 274, Fat 4.9, Fiber 8.5,

Carbs 40.8, Protein 19.2

7. Bacon and Cheese Crustless Quiche

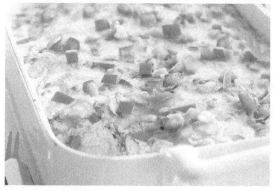

Preparation time: 10 minutes

Cooking Time: 4 hours

Servings: 6

Ingredients:

- 1 tablespoon butter
- 10 beaten eggs

- 8-ounces shredded cheddar cheese, reduced-fat
- 1 cup light cream
- ½ tablespoon black pepper
- 10 pieces chopped bacon, cooked

Directions:

1. Grease your slow cooker with butter and set aside.
2. Combine eggs, cheese, cream and pepper in a mixing bowl. Add mixture into the slow cooker.
3. Splash bacon over the mixture and cover the slow cooker.
4. Cook for about 4 hours on low. Make sure the quiche is not over-cooked.
5. Serve and enjoy.

Nutrition:

Calories: 436, Total fat: 36g,

Saturated fat: 16g, Total carbs: 4g,

Protein: 24g, Sugars: 1.6g, Fiber: 0.5g,

Sodium: 631mg, Potassium: 30.8g

8. Mushroom Crustless Quiche

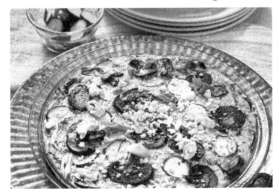

Preparation time: 15 minutes

Cooking Time: 4 hours

Servings: 6

Ingredients:

- 3 tablespoon butter, divided

- 1 package, 10-ounces, sliced mushrooms
- 1 red bell pepper, 1-inch strips
- ¼ tablespoon kosher salt
- 1 tablespoon minced onion, dried
- 10 beaten eggs
- ½ tablespoon black pepper
- 1 cup light cream
- 1 package, 10 ounces, shredded cheddar cheese, reduced fat

Directions:

1. Grease your slow cooker with 1 tablespoon butter.
2. Heat 2 tablespoon butter in a skillet for about 30 seconds over medium heat then add mushrooms, peppers, salt and onions.
3. Sauté for about 5 minutes until mushrooms lose water and pepper softens. Drain vegetables and transfer to the slow cooker.
4. Whisk together eggs, black pepper, cream, and cheese in a mixing bowl.
5. Add the egg mixture to vegetables into the slow cooker then stir to combine.
6. Cover the slow cooker and cook for about 4 hours on low. Make sure it's not to overcook.
7. Serve and enjoy

Nutrition:

Calories: 429,

Total fat: 35g,

Saturated fat: 20g,

Total carbs: 5.3g,

Protein: 23.2g,

Sugars: 2.7g,

Fiber: 0.9g,

Sodium: 738mg,

Potassium: 362mg

9. Maple Glazed Walnuts

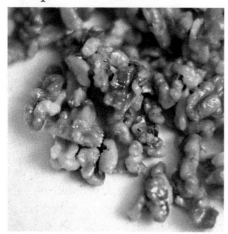

Preparation time: 15 minutes

Cooking time: 2 hours

Servings: 16

Ingredients:

- 16 oz walnuts
- ½ cup butter
- ½ cup maple syrup, sugar-free
- 1 tablespoon vanilla extract, pure

Directions:

1. *Add all the ingredients in the slow cooker and turn it to low.*
2. *Cook for 2 hours stirring occasionally to ensure all the nuts are well coated.*
3. *When the time has elapsed, transfer the walnuts onto a parchment paper. Let sit for some few minutes to cool.*
4. *Serve and enjoy.*

Nutrition:

Calories 328,

Total Fat 24g,

Saturated Fat 6g,

Total Carbs 10g,

Net Carbs 8g, Protein 4g,

Sugar: 7g, Fiber: 2g,

Sodium: 2mg,

Potassium 127g

10. Ham and Cheese Strata

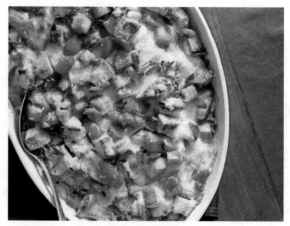

Preparation time: 10 minutes

Cooking time: 3 hours

Servings: 6

Ingredients:

- 1 tablespoon butter
- 8 slices low-carb Ezekiel bread divided into 16 triangles remove crust and save
- 6 oz thinly sliced ham, chopped
- 8 oz Monterey jack cheese, shredded,
- 2 tablespoon minced onions, dried
- 6 eggs
- 3 ¼ cups half-and-half
- ½ tablespoon salt
- ¼ tablespoon tabasco sauce
- ¾ tablespoon black pepper

Directions:

1. *Grease your slow cooker with butter then put 8 triangles of bread at the bottom. Sprinkle the trimmed off crust pieces to cover the bottom of your slow cooker with bread fully.*
2. *Sprinkle ham over the bread to make a thick layer, then add cheese preserving ½ cup.*
3. *Sprinkle half of the onions over cheese then top with remaining bread slices. Set aside.*

4. Mix eggs, half-and-half, salt, tabasco sauce and pepper in a mixing bowl until well blended.

5. Pour the egg mixture over bread then sprinkle remaining onions on top. Let sit for about 15 minutes.

6. Sprinkle preserved cheese and cover your slow cooker.

7. Cook for about 3 hours on low and when time has elapsed, uncover your slow cooker.

8. Let the strata sit for about 10 minutes before cutting.

9. Serve and enjoy.

Nutrition:

Calories: 481.4,

Total fat 37.8g,

Saturated fat 20.5g,

Total carbs 11.4g,

Protein 23.9g,

Sugar 1.1g,

Fiber 1g, Potassium 382mg,

Sodium 1334mg.

11. Breakfast Salad from Grains and Fruits

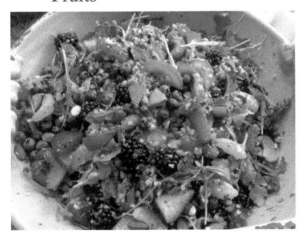

Preparation time: 5 minutes

Cooking time: 15 minutes

Servings: 6

Ingredients:

- 1 8-oz low fat vanilla yogurt
- 1 cup raisins
- 1 orange
- 1 Red delicious apple
- 1 Granny Smith apple
- ¾ cup bulgur
- ¾ cup quick cooking brown rice
- ¼ teaspoon salt
- 3 cups water

Direction:

1. On high fire, place a large pot and bring water to a boil.

2. Add bulgur and rice. Lower fire to a simmer and cooks for ten minutes while covered.

3. Turn off fire, set aside for 2 minutes while covered.

4. In baking sheet, transfer and evenly spread grains to cool.

5. Meanwhile, peel oranges and cut into sections. Chop and core apples.

6. Once grains are cool, transfer to a large serving bowl along with fruits.

7. Add yogurt and mix well to coat.

8. Serve and enjoy.

Nutrition:

Calories: 187;

Carbs: g;

Protein: g;

Fats: g;

Phosphorus: mg;

Potassium: mg;

Sodium: 117mg

12. French toast with Applesauce

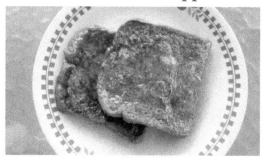

Preparation time: 5 minutes

Cooking time: 15 minutes

Servings: 6

Ingredients:

- ¼ cup unsweetened applesauce
- ½ cup milk
- 1 teaspoon ground cinnamon
- 2 eggs
- 2 tablespoon white sugar
- 6 slices whole wheat bread

Directions:

1. Mix well applesauce, sugar, cinnamon, milk and eggs in a mixing bowl.
2. Soak the bread, one by one into applesauce mixture until wet.
3. On medium fire, heat a nonstick skillet greased with cooking spray.
4. Add soaked bread one at a time and cook for 2-3 minutes per side or until lightly browned.
5. Serve and enjoy.

Nutrition:

Calories: 57;

Carbs: 6g;

Protein: 4g;

Fats: 4g;

Phosphorus: 69mg;

Potassium: 88mg;

Sodium: 43mg

13. Bagels Made Healthy

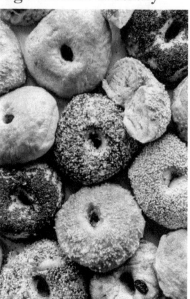

Preparation time: 5 minutes

Cooking time: 25 minutes

Servings: 8

Ingredients:

- 2 teaspoon yeast
- 1 ½ tablespoon olive oil
- 1 ¼ cups bread flour
- 2 cups whole wheat flour
- 1 tablespoon vinegar
- 2 tablespoon honey
- 1 ½ cups warm water

Directions:

1. In a bread machine, mix all ingredients, and then process on dough cycle.
2. Once done or end of cycle, create 8 pieces shaped like a flattened ball.
3. In the centre of each ball, make a hole using your thumb then create a donut shape.
4. In a greased baking sheet, place donut-shaped dough then covers and let it rise about ½ hour.
5. Prepare about 2 inches of water to boil in a large pan.

6. In a boiling water, drop one at a time the bagels and boil for 1 minute, then turn them once.

7. Remove them and return them to baking sheet and bake at 350oF (175oC) for about 20 to 25 minutes until golden brown.

Nutrition:

Calories: 221;

Carbs: 42g;

Protein: 7g;

Fats: g;

Phosphorus: 130mg;

Potassium: 166mg;

Sodium: 47mg

14. Cornbread with Southern Twist

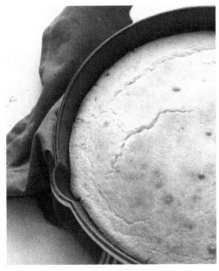

Preparation time: 15 minutes

Cooking time: 60 minutes

Servings: 8

Ingredients:

- 2 tablespoons shortening
- 1 ¼ cups skim milk
- ¼ cup egg substitute

- 4 tablespoons sodium free baking powder
- ½ cup flour
- 1 ½ cups cornmeal

Directions:

1. Prepare 8 x 8-inch baking dish or a black iron skillet then add shortening.

2. Put the baking dish or skillet inside the oven on 425oF, once the shortening has melted that means the pan is hot already.

3. In a bowl, add milk and egg then mix well.

4. Take out the skillet and add the melted shortening into the batter and stir well.

5. Pour all mixed ingredients into skillet.

6. For 15 to 20 minutes, cook in the oven until golden brown.

Nutrition:

Calories: 166;

Carbs: 35g;

Protein: 5g;

Fats: 1g;

Phosphorus: 79mg;

Potassium: 122mg;

Sodium: 34mg

15. Grandma's Pancake Special

Preparation time: 5 minutes

Cooking time: 15 minutes

Servings: 3

Ingredients:

- 1 tablespoon oil
- 1 cup milk
- 1 egg
- 2 teaspoons sodium free baking powder
- 2 tablespoons sugar
- 1 ¼ cups flour

Directions:

1. Mix all the dry ingredients such as the flour, sugar and baking powder.
2. Combine oil, milk and egg in another bowl. Once done, add them all to the flour mixture.
3. Make sure that as your stir the mixture, blend them until slightly lumpy.
4. In a hot greased griddle, pour-in at least ¼ cup of the batter to make each pancake.
5. To cook, ensure that the bottom is a bit brown, then turn and cook the other side, as well.

Nutrition:

Calories: 167;

Carbs: 50g;

Protein: 11g;

Fats: 11g;

Phosphorus: 176mg;

Potassium: 215mg;

Sodium: 70mg

16. Very Berry Smoothie

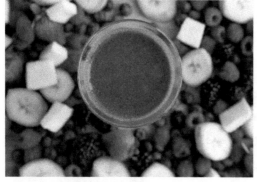

Preparation time: 3 minutes

Cooking time: 5 minutes

Servings: 2

Ingredients:

- 2 quarts water
- 2 cups pomegranate seeds

- 1 cup blackberries
- 1 cup blueberries

Directions:

1. Mix all ingredients in a blender.
2. Puree until smooth and creamy.
3. Transfer to a serving glass and enjoy.

Nutrition:

Calories: 464;

Carbs: 111g;

Protein: 8g;

Fats: 4g;

Phosphorus: 132mg;

Potassium: 843mg;

Sodium: 16mg

17. Pasta with Indian Lentils

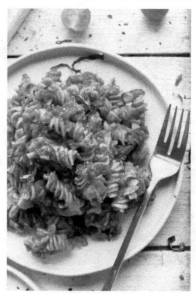

Preparation time: 5 minutes

Cooking time: 0 minutes

Servings: 6

Ingredients:

- ¼-½ cup fresh cilantro (chopped)
- 3 cups water
- 2 small dry red peppers (whole)
- 1 teaspoon turmeric

- 1 teaspoon ground cumin
- 2-3 cloves garlic (minced)
- 1 can (15 ounces) cubed tomatoes (with juice)
- 1 large onion (chopped)
- ½ cup dry lentils (rinsed)
- ½ cup orzo or tiny pasta

Directions:

1. In a skillet, combine all ingredients except for the cilantro then boil on medium-high heat.
2. Ensure to cover and slightly reduce heat to medium-low and simmer until pasta is tender for about 35 minutes.
3. Afterwards, take out the chili peppers then add cilantro and top it with low-fat sour cream.

Nutrition:

Calories: 175;

Carbs: 40g;

Protein: 3g;

Fats: 2g;

Phosphorus: 139mg;

Potassium: 513mg;

Sodium: 61mg

18. Pineapple Bread

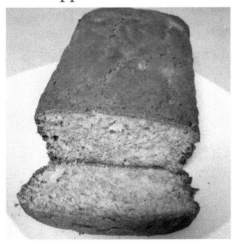

Preparation Time: 20 Minutes

Cooking Time: 1 Hour

Servings: 10

Ingredients:

- 1/3 cup Swerve
- 1/3 cup butter, unsalted
- 2 eggs
- 2 cups flour
- 3 teaspoons baking powder
- 1 cup pineapple, undrained
- 6 cherries, chopped

Directions:

1. Whisk the Swerve with the butter in a mixer until fluffy.
2. Stir in the eggs, then beat again.
3. Add the baking powder and flour, then mix well until smooth.
4. Fold in the cherries and pineapple.
5. Spread this cherry-pineapple batter in a 9x5 inch baking pan.
6. Bake the pineapple batter for 1 hour at 350 degrees F.
7. Slice the bread and serve.

Nutrition:

Calories 197,

Total Fat 7.2g,

Sodium 85mg,

Dietary Fiber 1.1g,

Sugars 3 g,

Protein 4g,

Calcium 79mg,

Phosphorous 316mg,

Potassium 227mg

19. Parmesan Zucchini Frittata

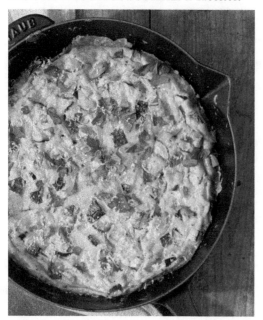

Preparation Time: 10 minutes

Cooking Time: 35 minutes

Servings: 6

Ingredients:

1 tablespoon olive oil

1 cup yellow onion, sliced

3 cups zucchini, chopped

½ cup Parmesan cheese, grated

8 large eggs

1/2 teaspoon black pepper

1/8 teaspoon paprika

3 tablespoons parsley, chopped

Directions:

Toss the zucchinis with the onion, parsley, and all other ingredients in a large bowl.

Pour this zucchini-garlic mixture in an 11x7 inches pan and spread it evenly.

Bake the zucchini casserole for approximately 35 minutes at 350 degrees F.

Cut in slices and serve.

Nutrition:

Calories 142,

Total Fat 9.7g,

Saturated Fat 2.8g,

Cholesterol 250mg,

Sodium 123mg,

Carbohydrate 4.7g,

Dietary Fiber 1.3g,

Sugars 2.4g,

Protein 10.2g,

Calcium 73mg,

Phosphorous 375mg,

Potassium 286mg

20. Texas Toast Casserole

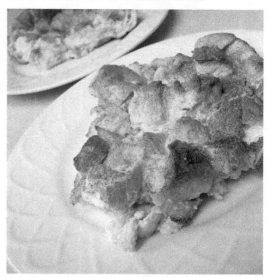

Preparation Time: 10 minutes

Cooking Time: 30 minutes

Servings: 10

Ingredients:

- 1/2 cup butter, melted
- 1 cup brown Swerve
- 1 lb. Texas Toast bread, sliced
- 4 large eggs
- 1 1/2 cup milk
- 1 tablespoon vanilla extract
- 2 tablespoons Swerve

- 2 teaspoons cinnamon
- Maple syrup for serving

Directions:

1. Layer a 9x13 inches baking pan with cooking spray.
2. Spread the bread slices at the bottom of the prepared pan.
3. Whisk the eggs with the remaining ingredients in a mixer.
4. Pour this mixture over the bread slices evenly.
5. Bake the bread for 30 minutes at 350 degrees F in a preheated oven.
6. Serve.

Nutrition:

Calories 332,

Total Fat 13.7g,

Sodium 350mg,

Dietary Fiber 2g,

Sugars 6g,

Protein 7.4g,

Calcium 143mg,

Phosphorous 186mg,

Potassium 74mg

CHAPTER 5:

Lunch Recipes

21. Salad with Vinaigrette

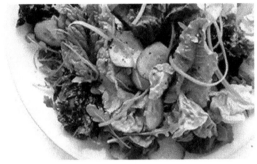

Preparation time: 25 minutes

Cooking time: 0 minutes

Servings: 4

Ingredients:

For the vinaigrette

- Olive oil – ½ cup
- Balsamic vinegar - 4 Tablespoons.
- Chopped fresh oregano – 2 Tablespoons.
- Pinch red pepper flakes
- Ground black pepper

For the salad

- Shredded green leaf lettuce – 4 cups
- Carrot – 1, shredded
- Fresh green beans – ¾ cup, cut into 1-inch pieces
- Large radishes – 3, sliced thin

Directions:

1. To make the vinaigrette: put the vinaigrette ingredients in a bowl and whisk.

2. To make the salad, in a bowl, toss together the carrot, lettuce, green beans, and radishes.

3. Add the vinaigrette to the vegetables and toss to coat.

4. Arrange the salad on plates and serve.

Nutrition:

Calories: 273 Fat: 27g Carb: 7g

Phosphorus: 30mg Potassium: 197mg

Sodium: 27mg Protein: 1g

22. Salad with Lemon Dressing

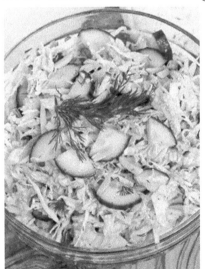

Preparation time: 10 minutes

Cooking time: 0 minutes

Servings: 4

Ingredients:

- Heavy cream – ¼ cup

- Freshly squeezed lemon juice – ¼ cup
- Granulated sugar – 2 Tablespoons.
- Chopped fresh dill – 2 Tablespoons.
- Finely chopped scallion – 2 Tablespoons. green part only
- Ground black pepper – ¼ teaspoon.
- English cucumber – 1, sliced thin
- Shredded green cabbage – 2 cups

Directions:

1. In a small bowl, stir together the lemon juice, cream, sugar, dill, scallion, and pepper until well blended.
2. In a large bowl, toss together the cucumber and cabbage.
3. Place the salad in the refrigerator and chill for 1 hour.
4. Stir before serving.

Nutrition:

Calories: 99 Fat: 6g

Carb: 13g Phosphorus: 38mg

Potassium: 200mg Sodium: 14mg Protein: 2g

23. Shrimp with Salsa

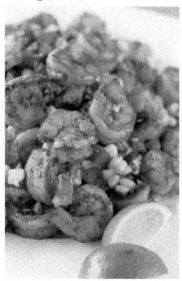

Preparation time: 15 minutes

Cooking time: 10 minutes

Servings: 4

Ingredients:

- Olive oil – 2 Tablespoon.
- Large shrimp – 6 ounces, peeled and deveined, tails left on
- Minced garlic – 1 teaspoon.
- Chopped English cucumber – ½ cup
- Chopped mango – ½ cup
- Zest of 1 lime
- Juice of 1 lime
- Ground black pepper
- Lime wedges for garnish

Directions:

1. Soak 4 wooden skewers in water for 30 minutes.
2. Preheat the barbecue to medium heat.
3. In a bowl, toss together the olive oil, shrimp, and garlic.
4. Thread the shrimp onto the skewers, about 4 shrimp per skewer.
5. In a bowl, stir together the mango, cucumber, lime zest, and lime juice, and season the salsa lightly with pepper. Set aside.
6. Grill the shrimp for 10 minutes, turning once or until the shrimp is opaque and cooked through.
7. Season the shrimp lightly with pepper.
8. Serve the shrimp on the cucumber salsa with lime wedges on the side.

Nutrition:

Calories: 120 Fat: 8g Carb: 4g

Phosphorus: 91mg Potassium: 129mg

Sodium: 60mg Protein: 9g

24. Cauliflower Soup

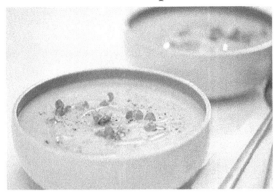

Preparation time: 30 minutes

Cooking time: 30 minutes

Servings: 6

Ingredients:

- Unsalted butter – 1 teaspoon.
- Sweet onion – 1 small, chopped
- Minced garlic – 2 teaspoons.
- Small head cauliflower – 1, cut into small florets
- Curry powder – 2 teaspoons.
- Water to cover the cauliflower
- Light sour cream – ½ cup
- Chopped fresh cilantro – 3 Tablespoons.

Directions:

1. In a large saucepan, heat the butter over a medium-high heat and sauté the onion-garlic for about 3 minutes or until softened.
2. Add the cauliflower, water, and curry powder.
3. Bring the soup to a boil, then reduce the heat to low and simmer for 20 minutes or until the cauliflower is tender.
4. Puree the soup until creamy and smooth with a hand mixer.
5. Transfer the soup back into a saucepan and stir in the sour cream and cilantro.

6. Heat the soup on medium heat for 5 minutes or until warmed through.

Nutrition:

Calories: 33

Fat: 2g

Carb: 4g

Phosphorus: 30mg

Potassium: 167mg

Sodium: 22mg

Protein: 1g

25. Cabbage Stew

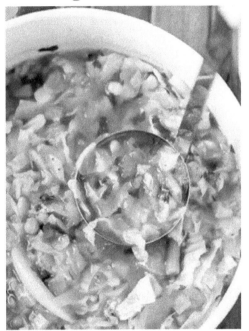

Preparation time: 20 minutes

Cooking time: 34 minutes

Servings: 6

Ingredients:

- Unsalted butter – 1 teaspoon.
- Large sweet onion - ½, chopped
- Minced garlic – 1 teaspoon.
- Shredded green cabbage – 6 cups
- Celery stalks - 3, chopped with leafy tops

- Scallion – 1, both green and white parts, chopped
- Chopped fresh parsley – 2 Tablespoons.
- Freshly squeezed lemon juice – 2 Tablespoons.
- Chopped fresh thyme – 1 Tablespoon.
- Chopped savory – 1 teaspoon.
- Chopped fresh oregano – 1 teaspoon.
- Water
- Fresh green beans – 1 cup, cut into 1-inch pieces
- Ground black pepper

Directions:

1. Melt the butter in a pot.
2. Sauté the onion and garlic in the melted butter for 3 minutes, or until the vegetables are softened.
3. Add the celery, cabbage, scallion, parsley, lemon juice, thyme, savory, and oregano to the pot, add enough water to cover the vegetables by 4 inches.
4. Bring the soup to a boil. Reduce the heat to low and simmer the soup for 25 minutes or until the vegetables are tender.
5. Add the green beans and simmer for 3 minutes.
6. Season with pepper.

Nutrition:

Calories: 33

Fat: 1g

Carb: 6g

Phosphorus: 29mg

Potassium: 187mg

Sodium: 20mg

Protein: 1g

26. Baked Haddock

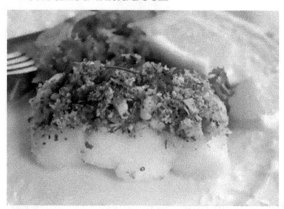

Preparation time: 10 minutes

Cooking time: 20 minutes

Servings: 4

Ingredients:

- Bread crumbs – ½ cup
- Chopped fresh parsley – 3 Tablespoons.
- Lemon zest – 1 Tablespoon.
- Chopped fresh thyme – 1 teaspoon.
- Ground black pepper – ¼ teaspoon.
- Melted unsalted butter – 1 Tablespoon.
- Haddock fillets – 12-ounces, deboned and skinned

Directions:

1. Preheat the oven to 350F.
2. In a bowl, stir together the parsley, breadcrumbs, lemon zest, thyme, and pepper until well combined.
3. Add the melted butter and toss until the mixture resembles coarse crumbs.
4. Place the haddock on a baking sheet and spoon the bread crumb mixture on top, pressing down firmly.
5. Bake the haddock in the oven for 20 minutes or until the fish is just cooked through and flakes off in chunks when pressed.

Nutrition:

Calories: 143

Fat: 4g

Carb: 10g

Phosphorus: 216mg

Potassium: 285mg

Sodium: 281mg

Protein: 16g

27. Herbed Chicken

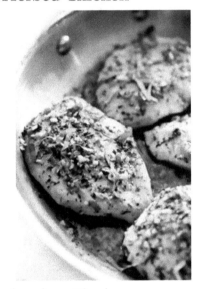

Preparation time: 20 minutes

Cooking time: 15 minutes

Servings: 4

Ingredients:

- Boneless, skinless chicken breast – 12 ounces, cut into 8 strips
- Egg white – 1
- Water – 2 Tablespoons. divided
- Breadcrumbs – ½ cup
- Unsalted butter – ¼ cup, divided
- Juice of 1 lemon
- Zest of 1 lemon
- Fresh chopped basil – 1 Tablespoon.
- Fresh chopped thyme – 1 teaspoon.
- Lemon slices, for garnish

Directions:

1. Place the chicken strips between 2 sheets of plastic wrap and pound each flat with a rolling pin.
2. In a bowl, whisk together the egg and 1 tablespoon. water.
3. Put the breadcrumbs in another bowl.
4. Dredge the chicken strips, one at a time, in the egg, then the breadcrumbs and set the breaded strips aside on a plate.
5. In a large skillet over medium heat, melt 2 tablespoons. Of the butter.
6. Cook the strips in the butter for 3 minutes, turning once, or until they are golden and cooked through. Transfer the chicken to a plate.
7. Add the lemon zest, lemon juice, basil, thyme, and remaining 1 tablespoon. Water to the skillet and stir until the mixture simmers.
8. Remove the sauce from the heat and stir in the remaining 2 tablespoons butter.
9. Serve the chicken with the lemon sauce drizzled over the top and garnished with lemon slices.

Nutrition:

Calories: 255

Fat: 14g

Carb: 11g

Phosphorus: 180mg

Potassium: 321mg

Sodium: 261mg

Protein: 20g

28. Pesto Pork Chops

Preparation time: 20 minutes

Cooking time: 20 minutes

Servings: 4

Ingredients:

- Pork top-loin chops – 4 (3-ounce) boneless, fat trimmed
- Herb pesto – 8 teaspoons.
- Breadcrumbs – ½ cup
- Olive oil – 1 Tablespoon.

Directions:

1. Preheat the oven to 450F.
2. Line a baking sheet with foil. Set aside.
3. Rub 1 teaspoon. of pesto evenly over both sides of each pork chop.
4. Lightly dredge each pork chop in the breadcrumbs.
5. Heat the oil in a skillet.
6. Brown the pork chops on each side for 5 minutes.
7. Place the pork chops on the baking sheet.
8. Bake for 10 minutes or until pork reaches 145F in the center.

Nutrition:

Calories: 210

Fat: 7g

Carb: 10g

Phosphorus: 179mg

Potassium: 220mg

Sodium: 148mg

Protein: 24g

29. Vegetable Curry

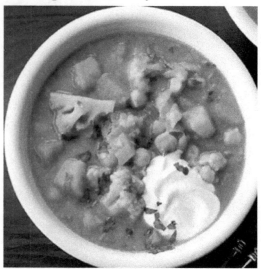

Preparation time: 15 minutes

Cooking time: 45 minutes

Servings: 4

Ingredients:

- Olive oil – 2 teaspoons.
- Sweet onion – ½, diced
- Minced garlic – 2 teaspoons.
- Grated fresh ginger – 2 teaspoons.
- Eggplant – ½, peeled and diced
- Carrot – 1, peeled and diced
- Red bell pepper – 1, diced
- Hot curry powder – 1 Tablespoon.
- Ground cumin – 1 teaspoon.
- Coriander – ½ teaspoon.
- Pinch cayenne pepper
- Homemade vegetable stock – 1 ½ cups
- Cornstarch – 1 Tablespoon.
- Water – ¼ cup

Directions:

1. Heat the oil in a stockpot.
2. Sauté the ginger, garlic, and onion for 3 minutes or until they are softened.

3. Add the red pepper, carrots, eggplant, and stir often for 6 minutes.

4. Stir in the cumin, curry powder, coriander, cayenne pepper, and vegetable stock.

5. Bring the curry to a boil and then lower the heat to low.

6. Simmer the curry for 30 minutes or until the vegetables are tender.

7. In a bowl, stir together the cornstarch and water.

8. Stir in the cornstarch mixture into the curry and simmer for 5 minutes or until the sauce has thickened.

Nutrition:

Calories: 100 Fat: 3g

Carb: 9g

Phosphorus: 28mg

Potassium: 180mg

Sodium: 218mg

Protein: 1g

30. Grilled Steak with Salsa

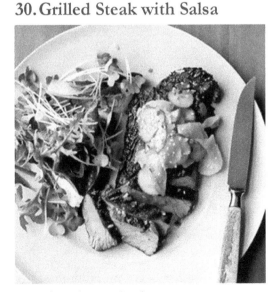

Preparation time: 20 minutes

Cooking time: 15 minutes

Servings: 4

Ingredients:

For the salsa

- Chopped English cucumber - 1 cup
- Boiled and diced red bell pepper – ¼ cup
- Scallion – 1, both green and white parts, chopped
- Chopped fresh cilantro – 2 Tablespoons.
- Juice of 1 lime

For the steak

- Beef tenderloin steaks – 4 (3-ounce), room temperature
- Olive oil
- Freshly ground black pepper

Directions:

1. In a bowl, to make the salsa, combine the lime juice, cilantro, scallion, bell pepper, and cucumber. Set aside.

2. To make the steak: Preheat a barbecue to medium heat.

3. Rub the steaks all over with oil and season with pepper.

4. Grill the steaks for about 5 minutes per side for medium-rare, or until the desired doneness.

5. Serve the steaks topped with salsa.

Nutrition:

Calories: 130

Fat: 6g

Carb: 1g

Phosphorus: 186mg

Potassium: 272mg

Sodium: 39mg

Protein: 19g

31. Buffalo Chicken Lettuce Wraps

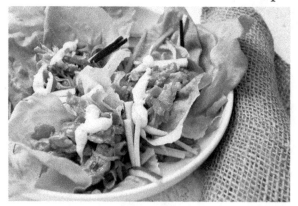

Preparation time: 10 minutes

Cooking time: 10 minutes

Servings: 4

Ingredients:

For the buffalo chicken filling

• Chicken tenderloin – 1 lb, cut into 1/2-inch cubes

• Vegetable oil – 3 tablespoons

• Crumbled blue cheese - 2/3 cup

• Light blue cheese dressing – ¼ cup

• Sour cream – ¼ cup.

• Hot pepper sauce

• Finely chopped celery – 2 stalks, trimmed

• Chopped fresh cilantro - 2 Tablespoons.

For the lettuce wraps

• Butterhead lettuce leaves – 8

• Celery sticks – 4, cut into smaller pieces

Directions:

1. To make the buffalo chicken filling:

2. In a bowl, combine the chicken, celery, hot pepper sauce, blue cheese, and sour cream.

3. Mix the ingredients with a spoon until well combined.

4. Cover the bowl and store in the refrigerator until ready to use.

5. To make the lettuce wraps:

6. Place the lettuce leaves on a platter or plate.

7. Divide the chicken mixture over the leaves and garnish with the celery sticks.

8. Serve the lettuce wraps cold or at room temperature.

Nutrition:

Calories: 106

Fat: 6g

Net Carbohydrates: 2g

Protein: 5g

Phosphorus: 216mg

Potassium: 285mg

Sodium: 281mg

Protein: 16g

32. Crazy Japanese Potato and Beef Croquettes

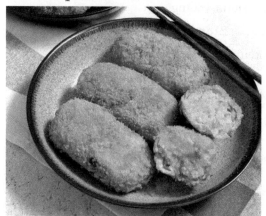

Preparation time: 10 minutes

Cooking Time: 20 minutes

Servings: 10

Ingredients:

• 3 medium russet potatoes, peeled and chopped

• 1 tablespoon almond butter

• 1 tablespoon vegetable oil

• 3 onions, diced

• ¾ pound ground beef

- 4 teaspoons light coconut aminos
- All-purpose flour for coating
- 2 eggs, beaten
- Panko bread crumbs for coating
- ½ cup oil, frying

Directions:

1. Take a saucepan and place it over medium-high heat; add potatoes and sunflower seeds water, boil for 16 minutes.
2. Remove water and put potatoes in another bowl, add almond butter and mash the potatoes.
3. Take a frying pan and place it over medium heat, add 1 tablespoon oil and let it heat up.
4. Add onions and stir fry until tender.
5. Add coconut aminos to beef to onions.
6. Keep frying until beef is browned.
7. Mix the beef with the potatoes evenly.
8. Take another frying pan and place it over medium heat; add half a cup of oil.
9. Form croquettes using the mashed potato mixture and coat them with flour, then eggs and finally breadcrumbs.
10. Fry patties until golden on all sides.

Nutrition:

Calories: 239

Fat: 4g

Carbohydrates: 20g

Protein: 10g

Phosphorus: 116mg

Potassium: 225mg

Sodium: 181mg

33. Saucy Garlic Greens

Preparation time: 5 minutes

Cooking Time: 20 minutes

Servings: 4

Ingredients:

- 1 bunch of leafy greens
- Sauce
- ½ cup cashews soaked in water for 10 minutes
- ¼ cup water
- 1 tablespoon lemon juice
- 1 teaspoon coconut aminos
- 1 clove peeled whole clove
- 1/8 teaspoon of flavored vinegar

Directions:

1. Make the sauce by draining and discarding the soaking water from your cashews and add the cashews to a blender.
2. Add fresh water, lemon juice, flavored vinegar, coconut aminos, garlic.
3. Blitz until you have a smooth cream and transfer to bowl.
4. Add ½ cup of water to the pot.
5. Place the steamer basket to the pot and add the greens in the basket.
6. Lock the lid and steam for 1 minute.
7. Quick-release the pressure.
8. Transfer the steamed greens to strainer and extract excess water.
9. Place the greens into a mixing bowl.
10. Add lemon garlic sauce and toss.

Nutrition:

Calories: 77 Fat: 5g Carbohydrates: 0g

Protein: 2g Phosphorus: 126mg

Potassium: 255mg

Sodium: 281mg

34. Garden Salad

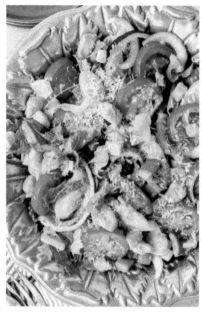

Preparation time: 5 minutes

Cooking Time: 20 minutes

Servings: 6

Ingredients:

- 1-pound raw peanuts in shell
- 1 bay leaf
- 2 medium-sized chopped up tomatoes
- ½ cup diced up green pepper
- ½ cup diced up sweet onion
- ¼ cup finely diced hot pepper
- ¼ cup diced up celery
- 2 tablespoons olive oil
- ¾ teaspoon flavored vinegar
- ¼ teaspoon freshly ground black pepper

Directions:

1. Boil your peanuts for 1 minute and rinse them.
2. The skin will be soft, so discard the skin.
3. Add 2 cups of water to the Instant Pot.
4. Add bay leaf and peanuts.
5. Lock the lid and cook on HIGH pressure for 20 minutes.
6. Drain the water.
7. Take a large bowl and add the peanuts, diced up vegetables.
8. Whisk in olive oil, lemon juice, pepper in another bowl.
9. Pour the mixture over the salad and mix.

Nutrition:

Calories: 140 Fat: 4g

Carbohydrates: 24g Protein: 5g

Phosphorus: 216mg Potassium: 185mg

Sodium: 141mg

35. Spicy Cabbage Dish

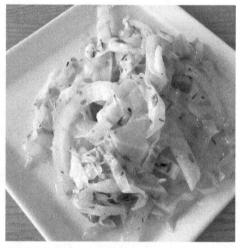

Preparation time: 10 minutes

Cooking Time: 4 hours

Servings: 4

Ingredients:

- 2 yellow onions, chopped
- 10 cups red cabbage, shredded
- 1 cup plums, pitted and chopped
- 1 teaspoon cinnamon powder
- 1 garlic clove, minced
- 1 teaspoon cumin seeds

- ¼ teaspoon cloves, ground
- 2 tablespoons red wine vinegar
- 1 teaspoon coriander seeds
- ½ cup water

Directions:

1. Add cabbage, onion, plums, garlic, cumin, cinnamon, cloves, vinegar, coriander and water to your Slow Cooker.
2. Stir well.
3. Place lid and cook on LOW for 4 hours.
4. Divide between serving platters.

Nutrition:

Calories: 197 Fat: 1g

Carbohydrates: 14g Protein: 3g

Phosphorus: 216mg Potassium: 285mg

Sodium: 281mg

36. Extreme Balsamic Chicken

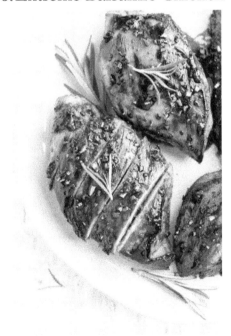

Preparation time: 10 minutes

Cooking Time: 35 minutes

Servings: 4

Ingredients:

- 3 boneless chicken breasts, skinless
- Sunflower seeds to taste
- ¼ cup almond flour
- 2/3 cups low-fat chicken broth
- 1 ½ teaspoons arrowroot
- ½ cup low sugar raspberry preserve
- 1 ½ tablespoons balsamic vinegar

Directions:

1. Cut chicken breast into bite-sized pieces and season them with seeds.
2. Dredge the chicken pieces in flour and shake off any excess.
3. Take a non-stick skillet and place it over medium heat.
4. Add chicken to the skillet and cook for 15 minutes, making sure to turn them half-way through.
5. Remove chicken and transfer to platter.
6. Add arrowroot, broth, raspberry preserve to the skillet and stir.
7. Stir in balsamic vinegar and reduce heat to low, stir-cook for a few minutes.
8. Transfer the chicken back to the sauce and cook for 15 minutes more.
9. Serve and enjoy!

Nutrition:

Calories: 546

Fat: 35g

Carbohydrates: 11g

Protein: 44g

Phosphorus: 136mg

Potassium: 195mg

Sodium: 81mg

37. Enjoyable Spinach and Bean Medley

Preparation time: 10 minutes

Cooking Time: 4 hours

Servings: 4

Ingredients:

- 5 carrots, sliced
- 1 ½ cups great northern beans, dried
- 2 garlic cloves, minced
- 1 yellow onion, chopped
- Pepper to taste
- ½ teaspoon oregano, dried
- 5 ounces baby spinach
- 4 ½ cups low sodium veggie stock
- 2 teaspoons lemon peel, grated
- 3 tablespoon lemon juice

Directions:

1. Add beans, onion, carrots, garlic, oregano and stock to your Slow Cooker.
2. Stir well.
3. Place lid and cook on HIGH for 4 hours.
4. Add spinach, lemon juice and lemon peel.
5. Stir and let it sit for 5 minutes.
6. Divide between serving platters and enjoy!

Nutrition:

Calories: 219

Fat: 8g

Carbohydrates: 14g

Protein: 8g

Phosphorus: 216mg

Potassium: 285mg

Sodium: 131mg

38. Tantalizing Cauliflower and Dill Mash

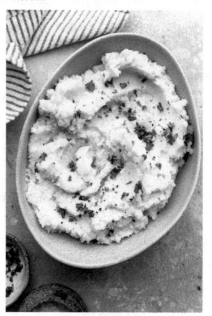

Preparation time: 10 minutes

Cooking Time: 6 hours

Servings: 6

Ingredients:

- 1 cauliflower head, florets separated
- 1/3 cup dill, chopped
- 6 garlic cloves
- 2 tablespoons olive oil
- Pinch of black pepper

Directions:

1. Add cauliflower to Slow Cooker.
2. Add dill, garlic and water to cover them.
3. Place lid and cook on HIGH for 5 hours. Drain the flowers.
4. Season with pepper and add oil, mash using potato masher.
5. Whisk and serve.

Nutrition:

Calories: 207 Fat: 4g Carbohydrates: 14g

Protein: 3g Phosphorus: 226mg

Potassium: 285mg Sodium: 134mg

39. Secret Asian Green Beans

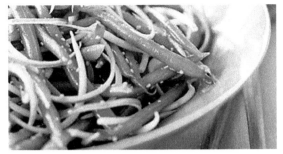

Preparation time: 10 minutes

Cooking Time: 2 hours

Servings: 10

Ingredients:

- 16 cups green beans, halved
- 3 tablespoons olive oil
- ¼ cup tomato sauce, salt-free
- ½ cup coconut sugar
- ¾ teaspoon low sodium soy sauce
- Pinch of pepper

Directions:

1. Add green beans, coconut sugar, pepper tomato sauce, soy sauce, oil to your Slow Cooker.
2. Stir well.
3. Place lid and cook on LOW for 3 hours.
4. Divide between serving platters and serve.
5. Enjoy!

Nutrition:

Calories: 200

Fat: 4g

Carbohydrates: 12g

Protein: 3g

Phosphorus: 216mg

Potassium: 285mg

Sodium: 131mg

40. Excellent Acorn Mix

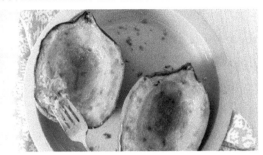

Preparation time: 10 minutes

Cooking Time: 7 hours

Servings: 10

Ingredients:

- 2 acorn squash, peeled and cut into wedges
- 16 ounces cranberry sauce, unsweetened
- ¼ teaspoon cinnamon powder
- Pepper to taste

Directions:

1. Add acorn wedges to your Slow Cooker.
2. Add cranberry sauce, cinnamon, raisins and pepper.
3. Stir.
4. Place lid and cook on LOW for 7 hours.
5. Serve and enjoy!

Nutrition:

Calories: 200

Fat: 3g

Carbohydrates: 15g

Protein: 2g

Phosphorus: 211mg

Potassium: 243mg

Sodium: 203mg

41. Crunchy Almond Chocolate Bars

Preparation time: 10 minutes

Cooking Time: 2 hours 30 minutes

Servings: 12

Ingredients:

- 1 egg white
- ¼ cup coconut oil, melted
- 1 cup coconut sugar
- ½ teaspoon vanilla extract
- 1 teaspoon baking powder
- 1 ½ cups almond meal
- ½ cup dark chocolate chips

Directions:

1. Take a bowl and add sugar, oil, vanilla extract, egg white, almond flour, baking powder and mix it well.
2. Fold in chocolate chips and stir.
3. Line Slow Cooker with parchment paper.
4. Grease.
5. Add the cookie mix and press on bottom.
6. Place lid and cook on LOW for 2 hours 30 minutes.
7. Take cookie sheet out and let it cool.
8. Cut in bars and enjoy!

Nutrition:

Calories: 200

Fat: 2g

Carbohydrates: 13g

Protein: 6g

Phosphorus: 136mg

Potassium: 285mg

Sodium: 281mg

42. Golden Eggplant Fries

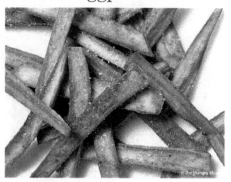

Preparation time: 10 minutes

Cooking Time: 15 minutes

Servings: 8

Ingredients:

- 2 eggs
- 2 cups almond flour
- 2 tablespoons coconut oil, spray
- 2 eggplant, peeled and cut thinly
- Sunflower seeds and pepper

Directions:

1. Preheat your oven to 400 degrees F.
2. Take a bowl and mix with sunflower seeds and black pepper.
3. Take another bowl and beat eggs until frothy.
4. Dip the eggplant pieces into the eggs.
5. Then coat them with the flour mixture.
6. Add another layer of flour and egg.
7. Then, take a baking sheet and grease with coconut oil on top.
8. Bake for about 15 minutes. Serve and enjoy!

Nutrition:

Calories: 212 Fat: 15.8g

Carbohydrates: 12.1g Protein: 8.6g

Phosphorus: 116mg Potassium: 185mg

Sodium: 121mg

43. Lettuce and Chicken Platter

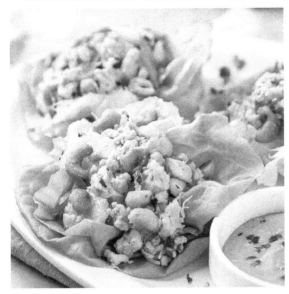

Preparation time: 10 minutes

Cooking Time: nil

Servings: 6

Ingredients:

- 2 cups chicken, cooked and coarsely chopped
- ½ head ice berg lettuce, sliced and chopped
- 1 celery rib, chopped
- 1 medium apple, cut
- ½ red bell pepper, deseeded and chopped
- 6-7 green olives, pitted and halved
- 1 red onion, chopped
- For dressing
- 1 tablespoon raw honey
- 2 tablespoons lemon juice
- Salt and pepper to taste

Directions:

1. Cut the vegetables and transfer them to your Salad Bowl.
2. Add olives.
3. Chop the cooked chicken and transfer to your Salad bowl.

4. Prepare dressing by mixing the ingredients listed under Dressing.
5. Pour the dressing into the Salad bowl.
6. Toss and enjoy!

Nutrition:

Calories: 296

Fat: 21g

Carbohydrates: 9g

Protein: 18g

Phosphorus: 146mg

Potassium: 205mg

Sodium: 221mg

44. Greek Lemon Chicken Bowl

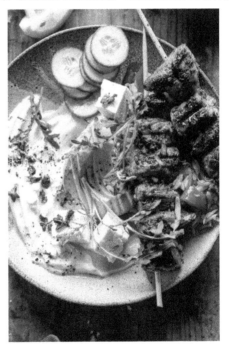

Preparation time: 10 minutes

Cooking Time: 15 minutes

Servings: 6

Ingredients:

- 2 cups chicken, cooked and chopped
- 2 cans chicken broth, fat free

- 2 medium carrots, chopped
- ¼ teaspoon pepper
- 2 tablespoons parsley, snipped
- ¼ cup lemon juice
- 1 can cream chicken soup, fat free, low sodium
- ½ cup onion, chopped
- 1 garlic clove, minced

Directions:

1. Take a pot and add all the ingredients except parsley into it.
2. Season with salt and pepper.
3. Bring the mix to a boil over medium-high heat.
4. Reduce the heat and simmer for 15 minutes.
5. Garnish with parsley.
6. Serve hot and enjoy!

Nutrition:

Calories: 520 Fat: 33g

Carbohydrates: 31g Protein: 30g

Phosphorus: 216mg Potassium: 285mg

Sodium: 281mg

45. Spicy Chili Crackers

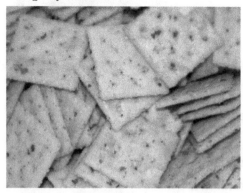

Preparation time: 15 minutes

Cooking Time: 60 minutes

Servings: 10

Ingredients:

- ¾ cup almond flour
- ¼ cup coconut four
- ¼ cup coconut flour
- ½ teaspoon paprika
- ½ teaspoon cumin
- 1 ½ teaspoons chili pepper spice
- 1 teaspoon onion powder
- ½ teaspoon sunflower seeds
- 1 whole egg
- ¼ cup unsalted almond butter

Directions:

1. Preheat your oven to 350 degrees F.
2. Line a baking sheet with parchment paper and keep it on the side.
3. Add ingredients to your food processor and pulse until you have a nice dough.
4. Divide dough into two equal parts.
5. Place one ball on a sheet of parchment paper and cover with another sheet; roll it out.
6. Cut into crackers and repeat with the other ball.
7. Transfer the prepped dough to a baking tray and bake for 8-10 minutes.
8. Remove from oven and serve.
9. Enjoy!

Nutrition:

Total Carbs: 2.8g

Fiber: 1g

Protein: 1.6g

Fat: 4.1g

Phosphorus: 216mg

Potassium: 285mg

Sodium: 191mg

46. Dolmas Wrap

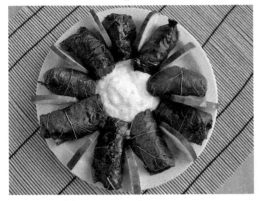

Preparation Time: 10 minutes

Cooking time: 10 minutes

Servings: 2

Ingredients:

- 2 whole wheat wrap
- 6 dolmas (stuffed grape leaves)
- 1 tomato, chopped
- 1 cucumber, chopped
- 2 oz Greek yogurt
- ½ teaspoon minced garlic
- ¼ cup lettuce, chopped
- 2 oz Feta, crumbled

Directions:

1. In the mixing bowl combine together chopped tomato, cucumber, Greek yogurt, minced garlic, lettuce, and Feta.
2. When the mixture is homogenous transfer it in the center of every wheat wrap.
3. Arrange dolma over the vegetable mixture.
4. Carefully wrap the wheat wraps.

Nutrition:

Calories 341,

Fat 12.9,

Fiber 9.2,

Carbs 52.4,

Protein 13.2

Phosphorus: 206mg

Potassium: 125mg

Sodium: 181mg

47. Green Palak Paneer

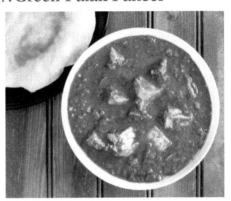

Preparation time: 5 minutes

Cooking Time: 10 minutes

Servings: 4

Ingredients:

- 1-pound spinach
- 2 cups cubed paneer (vegan)
- 2 tablespoons coconut oil
- 1 teaspoon cumin
- 1 chopped up onion
- 1-2 teaspoons hot green chili minced up
- 1 teaspoon minced garlic
- 15 cashews
- 4 tablespoons almond milk
- 1 teaspoon Garam masala
- Flavored vinegar as needed

Directions:

1. Add cashews and milk to a blender and blend well.
2. Set your pot to Sauté mode and add coconut oil; allow the oil to heat up.

3. Add cumin seeds, garlic, green chilies, ginger and sauté for 1 minute.

4. Add onion and sauté for 2 minutes.

5. Add chopped spinach, flavored vinegar and a cup of water.

6. Lock up the lid and cook on HIGH pressure for 10 minutes.

7. Quick-release the pressure.

8. Add ½ cup of water and blend to a paste. Add cashew paste, paneer and Garam Masala and stir thoroughly.

9. Serve over hot rice!

Nutrition:

Calories: 367 Fat: 26g

Carbohydrates: 21g Protein: 16g

Phosphorus: 236mg Potassium: 385mg

Sodium: 128mg

48. Sporty Baby Carrots

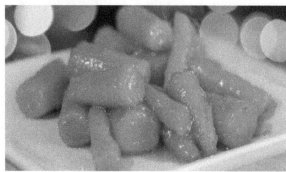

Preparation time: 5 minutes

Cooking Time: 5 minutes

Servings: 4

Ingredients:

- 1-pound baby carrots
- 1 cup water
- 1 tablespoon clarified ghee
- 1 tablespoon chopped up fresh mint leaves
- Sea flavored vinegar as needed

Directions:

1. Place a steamer rack on top of your pot and add the carrots.

2. Add water. Lock the lid and cook at HIGH pressure for 2 minutes.

3. Do a quick release.

4. Pass the carrots through a strainer and drain them.

5. Wipe the insert clean.

6. Return the insert to the pot and set the pot to Sauté mode.

7. Add clarified butter and allow it to melt. Add mint and sauté for 30 seconds. Add carrots to the insert and sauté well. Remove them and sprinkle with bit of flavored vinegar on top.

Nutrition:

Calories: 131 Fat: 10g Sodium: 81mg

Carbohydrates: 11g Protein: 1g

Phosphorus: 116mg Potassium: 185mg

49. Traditional Black Bean Chili

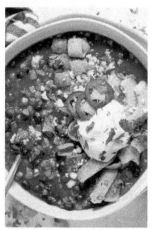

Preparation time: 10 minutes

Cooking Time: 4 hours

Servings: 4

Ingredients:

- 1 ½ cups red bell pepper, chopped

- 1 cup yellow onion, chopped
- 1 ½ cups mushrooms, sliced
- 1 tablespoon olive oil
- 1 tablespoon chili powder
- 2 garlic cloves, minced
- 1 teaspoon chipotle chili pepper, chopped
- ½ teaspoon cumin, ground
- 16 ounces canned black beans, drained and rinsed
- 2 tablespoons cilantro, chopped
- 1 cup tomatoes, chopped

Directions:

1. Add red bell peppers, onion, dill, mushrooms, chili powder, garlic, chili pepper, cumin, black beans, and tomatoes to your Slow Cooker.
2. Stir well.
3. Place lid and cook on HIGH for 4 hours.
4. Sprinkle cilantro on top.
5. Serve and enjoy!

Nutrition:

Calories: 211 Fat: 3g Sodium: 201mg

Carbohydrates: 22g Protein: 5g

Phosphorus: 216mg Potassium: 245mg

50. Very Wild Mushroom Pilaf

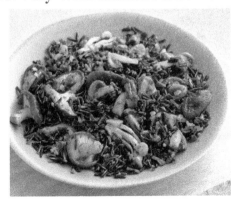

Preparation time: 10 minutes

Cooking Time: 3 hours

Servings: 4

Ingredients:

- 1 cup wild rice
- 2 garlic cloves, minced
- 6 green onions, chopped
- 2 tablespoons olive oil
- ½ pound baby Bella mushrooms
- 2 cups water

Directions:

1. Add rice, garlic, onion, oil, mushrooms and water to your Slow Cooker.
2. Stir well until mixed.
3. Place lid and cook on LOW for 3 hours.
4. Stir pilaf and divide between serving platters.
5. Enjoy!

Nutrition:

Calories: 210 Fat: 7g

Carbohydrates: 16g

Protein: 4g

Phosphorus: 266mg

Potassium: 232mg

Sodium: 176mg

51. Chilled Chicken, Artichoke and Zucchini Platter

Preparation time: 10 minutes

Cooking Time: 5 minutes

Servings: 4

Ingredients:

- 2 medium chicken breasts, cooked and cut into 1-inch cubes
- ¼ cup extra virgin olive oil

- 2 cups artichoke hearts, drained and roughly chopped

- 3 large zucchinis, diced/cut into small rounds

- 1 can (15 ounce) chickpeas

- 1 cup Kalamata olives

- ½ teaspoon Fresh ground black pepper

- ½ teaspoon Italian seasoning

- ¼ cup parmesan, grated

Directions:

1. Take a large skillet and place it over medium heat, heat olive oil.

2. Add zucchini and sauté for 5 minutes, season with salt and pepper.

3. Remove from heat and add all the listed ingredients to the skillet.

4. Stir until combined.

5. Transfer to glass container and store.

6. Serve and enjoy!

Nutrition:

Calories: 457

Fat: 22g

Carbohydrates: 30g

Protein: 24g

Phosphorus: 216mg

Potassium: 285mg

Sodium: 157mg

52. Chicken and Carrot Stew

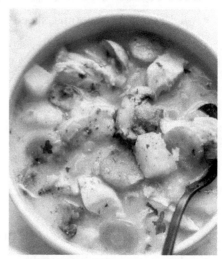

Preparation time: 15 minutes

Cooking Time: 6 hours

Servings: 6

Ingredients:

- 4 chicken breasts, boneless and cubed

- 2 cups chicken broth

- 1 cup tomatoes, chopped

- 3 cups carrots, peeled and cubed

- 1 teaspoon thyme dried

- 1 cup onion, chopped

- 2 garlic cloves, minced

- Pepper to taste

Directions:

1. Add all the ingredients to the Slow Cooker.

2. Stir and close the lid.

3. Cook for 6 hours.

4. Serve hot and enjoy!

Nutrition:

Calories: 182 Fat: 4g

Carbohydrates: 10g Protein: 39g

Phosphorus: 216mg

Potassium: 285mg

Sodium: 212mg

53. Tasty Spinach Pie

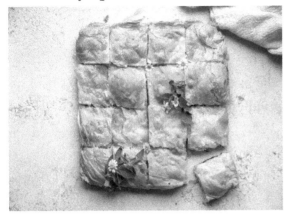

Preparation time: 10 minutes

Cooking Time: 4 hours

Servings: 2

Ingredients:

- 10 ounces spinach
- 2 cups baby Bella mushrooms, chopped
- 1 red bell pepper, chopped
- 1 ½ cups low-fat cheese, shredded
- 8 whole eggs
- 1 cup coconut cream
- 2 tablespoons chives, chopped
- Pinch of pepper
- ½ cup almond flour
- ¼ teaspoon baking soda

Directions:

1. Take a bowl and add eggs, coconut cream, chives, pepper and whisk well.
2. Add almond flour, baking soda, cheese, mushrooms bell pepper, spinach and toss well.
3. Grease your cooker and transfer mix to the Slow Cooker.
4. Place lid and cook on LOW for 4 hours.
5. Slice and enjoy!

Nutrition:

Calories: 201

Fat: 6g

Carbohydrates: 8g

Protein: 5g

Phosphorus: 216mg

Potassium: 275mg

Sodium: 121mg

54. Mesmerizing Carrot and Pineapple Mix

Preparation time: 10 minutes

Cooking Time: 6 hours

Servings: 10

Ingredients:

- 1 cup raisins
- 6 cups water
- 23 ounces natural applesauce
- 2 tablespoons stevia
- 2 tablespoons cinnamon powder
- 14 ounces carrots, shredded
- 8 ounces canned pineapple, crushed
- 1 tablespoon pumpkin pie spice

Directions:

1. Add carrots, applesauce, raisins, stevia, cinnamon, pineapple, pumpkin pie spice to your Slow Cooker and gently stir.
2. Place lid and cook on LOW for 6 hours.
3. Serve and enjoy!

Nutrition:

Calories: 179 Fat: 5g

Carbohydrates: 15g Protein: 4g

Phosphorus: 216mg Potassium: 285mg

Sodium: 134mg

55. Blackberry Chicken Wings

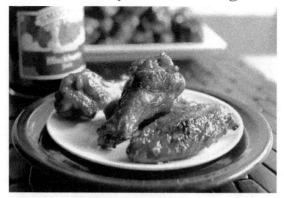

Preparation time: 35 minutes

Cooking Time: 50minutes

Servings: 4

Ingredients:

- 3 pounds chicken wings, about 20 pieces
- ½ cup blackberry chipotle jam
- Sunflower seeds and pepper to taste
- ½ cup water

Directions:

1. Add water and jam to a bowl and mix well.
2. Place chicken wings in a zip bag and add two-thirds of the marinade.
3. Season with sunflower seeds and pepper.
4. Let it marinate for 30 minutes.
5. Pre-heat your oven to 400 degrees F.
6. Prepare a baking sheet and wire rack, place chicken wings in wire rack and bake for 15 minutes.
7. Brush remaining marinade and bake for 30 minutes more.
8. Enjoy!

Nutrition:

Calories: 502 Fat: 39g Carbohydrates: 01.8g

Protein: 34g Phosphorus: 216mg

Potassium: 305mg Sodium: 131mg

56. Generous   Lemon   Dredged Broccoli

Preparation time: 10 minutes

Cooking Time: 15 minutes

Servings: 4

Ingredients:

- 2 heads broccoli, separated into florets
- 2 teaspoons extra virgin olive oil
- 1 teaspoon sunflower seeds
- ½ teaspoon pepper
- 1 garlic clove, minced
- ½ teaspoon lemon juice

Directions:

1. Pre-heat your oven to a temperature of 400 degrees F.
2. Take a large sized bowl and add broccoli florets with some extra virgin olive oil, pepper, sea sunflower seeds and garlic.
3. Spread the broccoli out in a single even layer on a fine baking sheet.
4. Bake in your pre-heated oven for about 15-20 minutes until the florets are soft enough to be pierced with a fork.
5. Squeeze lemon juice over them generously before serving.
6. Enjoy!

Nutrition:

Calories: 49

Fat: 2g

Carbohydrates: 4g

Protein: 3g

Phosphorus: 216mg

Potassium: 285mg

Sodium: 141mg

57. Tantalizing Almond butter Beans

Preparation time: 5 minutes

Cooking Time: 12 minutes

Servings: 4

Ingredients:

- 2 garlic cloves, minced
- Red pepper flakes to taste
- Sunflower seeds to taste
- 2 tablespoons clarified butter
- 4 cups green beans, trimmed

Directions:

1. Bring a pot of water to boil, with added seeds for taste.
2. Once the water starts to boil, add beans and cook for 3 minutes.
3. Take a bowl of ice water and drain beans, plunge them into the ice water.
4. Once cooled, keep them on the side.
5. Take a medium skillet and place it over medium heat, add ghee and melt.
6. Add red pepper, sunflower seeds, garlic.
7. Cook for 1 minute.
8. Add beans and toss until coated well, cook for 3 minutes.
9. Serve and enjoy!

Nutrition:

Calories: 93

Fat: 8g

Carbohydrates: 4g

Protein: 2g

Phosphorus: 316mg

Potassium: 225mg

Sodium: 189mg

58. Healthy Chicken Cream Salad

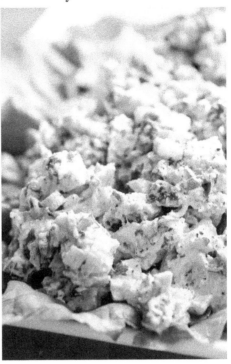

Preparation time: 5 minutes

Cooking Time: 50 minutes

Servings: 3

Ingredients:

- 2 chicken breasts
- 1 ½ cups low fat cream
- 3 ounces celery
- 2-ounce green pepper, chopped
- ½ ounce green onion, chopped
- ½ cup low fat mayo
- 3 hard-boiled eggs, chopped

Directions:

1. Pre-heat your oven to 350 degrees F.
2. Take a baking sheet and place chicken, cover with cream.
3. Bake for 30-40 minutes.
4. Take a bowl and mix in the chopped celery, peppers, onions.
5. Chop the baked chicken into bite-sized portions.

6. Peel and chop the hard-boiled eggs.

7. Take a large salad bowl and mix in eggs, veggies and chicken.

8. Toss well and serve.

Nutrition:

Calories: 415 Fat: 24g Carbohydrates: 4g

Protein: 40g Phosphorus: 216mg

Potassium: 212mg Sodium: 141mg

59. Generously Smothered Pork Chops

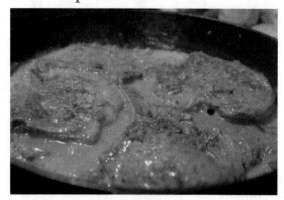

Preparation time: 10 minutes

Cooking Time: 30 minutes

Servings: 4

Ingredients:

- 4 pork chops, bone-in
- 2 tablespoons of olive oil
- ¼ cup vegetable broth
- ½ pound Yukon gold potatoes, peeled and chopped
- 1 large onion, sliced
- 2 garlic cloves, minced
- 2 teaspoon rubbed sage
- 1 teaspoon thyme, ground
- Pepper as needed

Directions:

1. Pre-heat your oven to 350 degrees F.

2. Take a large sized skillet and place it over medium heat.

3. Add a tablespoon of oil and allow the oil to heat up.

4. Add pork chops and cook them for 4-5 minutes per side until browned.

5. Transfer chops to a baking dish.

6. Pour broth over the chops.

7. Add remaining oil to the pan and sauté potatoes, onion, garlic for 3-4 minutes.

8. Take a large bowl and add potatoes, garlic, onion, thyme, sage, pepper.

9. Transfer this mixture to the baking dish (wish pork).

10. Bake for 20-30 minutes.

11. Serve and enjoy!

Nutrition:

Calorie: 261 Fat: 10g Carbohydrates: 1.3g

Protein: 2g Phosphorus: 196mg

Potassium: 285mg Sodium: 111mg

60. Caramel Apple Salad

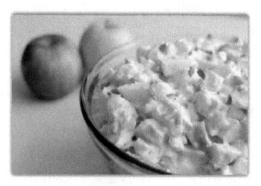

Preparation time: 10 minutes

Cooking time: 0 minutes

Servings: 4

Ingredients:

- 3 cups apples, chopped
- 8 ounces canned crushed pineapple
- 8 ounces whipped topping

- ½ cup butterscotch topping
- 1/3 cup peanuts
- ¼ cup butterscotch chips

Directions:

1. Throw all the salad ingredients into a suitably-sized salad bowl.
2. Toss them well and refrigerate for 1 hour.
3. Serve.

Nutrition:

Calories: 196 Protein: 1 g

Carbohydrates: 30 g Fat: 8 g

Cholesterol: 0 mg Sodium: 37 mg

Potassium: 105 mg Phosphorus: 47 mg

Calcium: 13 mg Fiber: 1.3 g

61. Chicken and Veggie Soup

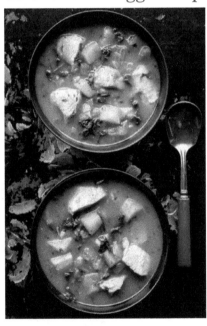

Preparation Time: 15minutes

Cooking Time: 25minutes

Servings: 8

Ingredients:

- 4 cups cooked and chopped chicken
- 7 cups reduced-sodium chicken broth

- 1 pound frozen white corn
- 1 medium onion diced
- 4 - Cloves garlic minced
- 2 - Carrots peeled and diced
- 2 - Celery stalks chopped
- 2 - Teaspoons oregano
- 2 - Teaspoon curry powder
- ½ - teaspoon black pepper

Directions:

1. Include all fixings into the moderate cooker.
2. Cook on LOW for 8hrs.
3. Serve over cooked white rice.

Nutrition:

Calories220 Fat: 7g Protein: 24g Carbs: 19g

62. Pesto Chicken

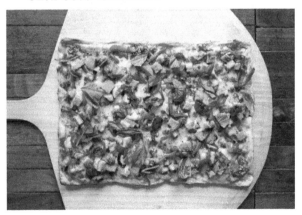

Preparation Time: 5minutes

Cooking Time: 30minutes

Servings: 6

Ingredients:

- 3 - Chicken breast fillets
- 6 - Ounce jar of pesto
- ½ - cup of reduced-sodium chicken

Directions:

1. Spot chicken bosoms at the base of the moderate cooker.

2. Pour pesto over the chicken and spread to coat the highest points of the chicken.

3. Pour in ½ cup chicken stock.

4. Cook on LOW for 6 to 8hrs.

5. Serve over cooked pasta.

Nutrition:

Calories: 278

Fat: 18g

Protein: 28g

Carbs: 1g

63. Spicy Coconut Curry Chicken

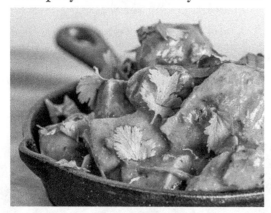

Preparation Time: 20minutes

Cooking Time: 50minutes

Servings: 4

Ingredients:

- 2 - Boneless chicken breasts (fresh or frozen)

- ¼ - cup chopped green onions

- 1 - (4 ounce) diced green chili peppers

- 2 - Tablespoons minced garlic

- 1 ½ - Tablespoons curry powder

- 1 - Tablespoon chili powder

- 1 - teaspoon cumin

- ½ - teaspoon cinnamon

- 1 - Tablespoon lime juice

- 1 ½ - cup water

- 1 - (7 ounce) can coconut milk

- 1 - cup dry white rice

- Chopped cilantro, for garnish

Directions:

1. Consolidate all fixings except for coconut milk and rice in the moderate cooker.

2. Spread and cook on LOW for 7-9hrs.

3. In the wake of cooking time, shred chicken with a fork, mix in coconut milk and dry rice.

4. Turn the moderate cooker to HIGH and cook for an extra 30mins, or until the rice has consumed the fluid and is cooked.

5. Serve hot and decorate with cilantro.

Nutrition:

Calories: 270 Fat: 19g Protein: 20g Carbs: 7g

64. Chicken Enchilada Casserole

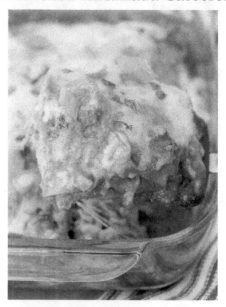

Preparation Time: 30mins

Cooking Time: 45mins

Servings: 8

Ingredients:

- 9 - Corn tortillas, 6-inch

- 2 - Cups cooked diced chicken
- 1 to 16 - ounce bag frozen corn
- 1 - Teaspoon chili powder
- ¼ - teaspoon ground black pepper
- 1 - Can (4 ounces) chopped green chili peppers, mild
- 1 - cup shredded Mexican blend cheese
- 1 - Cup green chili salsa
- 1 - can (15 ounces) no sodium black beans, rinsed and drained,
- ½ - cup sour cream

Directions:

1. Splash moderate cooker with cooking shower. Spot 3 tortillas in the base of the moderate range.
2. Top tortillas with half of the chicken, the corn, about portion of the seasonings, and half of the stew peppers.
3. Sprinkle with half of the destroyed cheddar and pour about ½ cup salsa over the cheddar.
4. Rehash with 3 additional tortillas, the dark beans, staying chicken, seasonings, stew peppers, and cheddar.
5. Top with great tortillas and salsa.
6. Spread and cook on LOW for 5 to 6hrs.
7. Serve warm and can include one Tablespoon of acrid cream on each plate.

Nutrition:

Calories: 308

Fat: 10g

Protein: 20g

Carbs: 37g

65. Orange Chicken

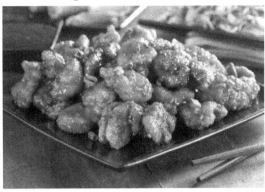

Preparation Time: 10mins

Cooking Time: 13mins

Servings: 8

Ingredients:

- 8 - bone-in chicken thighs
- 1/3 - cup flour
- 1 - Tablespoon balsamic vinegar
- 1 - Tablespoon ketchup
- 4 - Ounces orange juice
- 1 - Tablespoon brown sugar
- 1 - Medium onion, chopped
- Medium bell pepper, chopped

Directions:

1. Spot chicken and flour into a plastic sack, shake to coat.
2. Add covered chicken to the moderate cooker.
3. Blend the squeezed orange, dark colored sugar, vinegar, and ketchup into a bowl.
4. Pour sauce into the moderate cooker over the chicken and blend.
5. Cook on LOW 6 to 8hrs.
6. Draw chicken off of the bone and serve over white rice with a portion of the sauce.

Nutrition:

Calories: 236 Fat: 15g Protein: 17g

Carbs: 8.4g

66. Balsamic Chicken Thighs

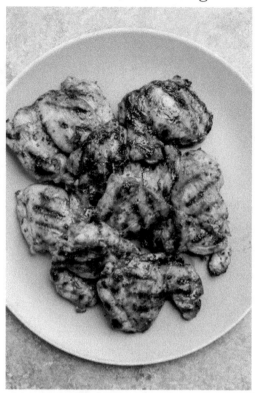

Preparation Time: 15mins

Cooking Time: 20mins

Servings: 8

Ingredients:

- 8 - Chicken thighs
- 1 - Teaspoon garlic powder
- 1 - teaspoon dried basil
- ½ - teaspoon salt
- ½ - teaspoon pepper
- 2 - teaspoons dried minced onion
- 4 - garlic cloves, minced
- 1 - Tablespoon olive oil
- ½ - cup balsamic vinegar
- Fresh chopped parsley

Directions:

1. Join the initial 5 dry flavors in a touch bowl and unfold over chicken on the 2 aspects. Put in a secure spot.
2. Pour olive oil and garlic on the base of the moderate cooker.
3. Spot hen on top.
4. Pour balsamic vinegar over the bird.
5. Spread and cook dinner on LOW for 6 to 8hrs.
6. Sprinkle with crisp parsley on top. Serve over noodles.

Nutrition:

Calories: 230

Fat: 16g

Protein: 16g

Carbs: 3g

67. Honey Sesame Chicken

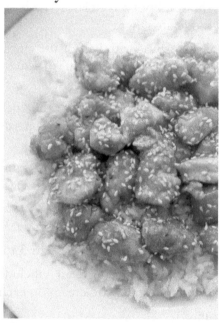

Preparation Time: 10mins

Cook Time: 15mins

Servings: 6

Ingredients:

- 6 - skinless chicken thighs
- 1 - Tablespoon olive oil
- ½ - cup honey
- 2 - Tablespoon sesame seeds

- ¼ - cup light low sodium soy sauce
- ¼ - cup water
- 1 - Tablespoon sesame oil
- 1 - teaspoon pepper
- 1 (10 ounces) package frozen broccoli

Directions:

1. Spot all fixings in a cooler sack, toss to coat.
2. Spot in the moderate cooker and cook on LOW for 4 to 5hrs.
3. Take chicken and shred, and after that arrival to the sauce.
4. Serve over hot cooked rice.

Nutrition:

Calories: 247

Fat: 9g

Protein: 16g

Carbs: 28g

68. Hawaiian Chicken and Rice

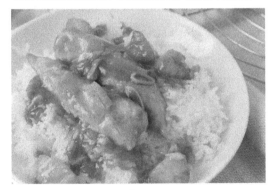

Preparation Time: 15mins

Cooking Time: 20mins

Servings: 11

Ingredients:

- 6 - inch piece ginger, chopped into 1 - inch pieces
- 2 - medium carrots, chopped into ½ - inch pieces

- 2 - cup uncooked white rice, rinsed
- 1 - pound boneless skinless chicken thighs
- 7 - cups no/low sodium chicken broth
- 1 - Tablespoon oyster flavored sauce
- 1 - Tablespoon low sodium soy sauce
- 1 - Tablespoon sesame oil
- 1 - small green cabbage, chopped into bite-sized pieces
- 12 - medium green onions, chopped into 1 - inch pieces
- Cilantro

Directions:

1. Refrigerate hacked cabbage, green onions, and Chinese parsley (discretionary) until prepared to utilize.
2. In moderate cooker, consolidate ginger, carrots, rice, chicken, and spread with chicken soup.
3. Spread moderate cooker and cook on LOW for 7 to 9hrs.
4. During the last 1hr of cooking, open the moderate cooker and blend in cabbage and green onions. Spread and cook for 60 minutes.
5. Include shellfish sauce, soy sauce, cilantro, and sesame oil into the pot before serving.
6. Present with canned pineapple whenever wanted

Nutrition:

Calories: 371

Fat: 6g

Protein: 25g

Carbs: 54g

69. Shredded Chicken Taco Filling

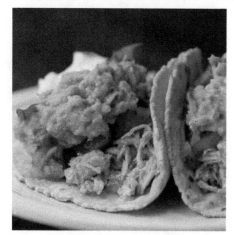

Preparation Time: 15mins

Cooking Time: 15mins

Servings: 10

Ingredients:

- 2 - cups diced onions
- 2 ¼ - pounds boneless, skinless chicken breast
- ½ - cup lime juice
- 1 - teaspoon ground coriander
- 2 ½ - teaspoons cumin
- 2 - teaspoons garlic powder
- 1 - Tablespoon smoked paprika
- 1 ½ - teaspoon chili powder

Directions:

1. With cooking oil try spray the side and bottom of a cooker.
2. Spot onions on the base of the slight cooker; include chicken, lime squeeze and flavors. Cook on LOW for 8hrs or until the hen is completed;
3. Shred chook with 2 forks.
4. It can serve on flour tortillas and top with lettuce and sharp cream (optional).

Nutrition:

Calories: 117 Fat: 3g Protein: 22g Carbs: 5g

70. Mexican Beef Flour Wrap

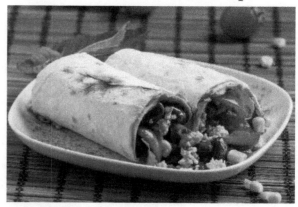

Preparation Time: 10 minutes

Cooking Time: 10 minutes

Servings: 2

Ingredients:

- 5 oz. Cooked roast beef
- 8 cucumber slices
- 2 flour tortillas, 6-inch size
- 2 tbsp. Whipped cream cheese
- 2 leaves light green lettuce
- 1/4 bowl cut red onion
- 1/4 stripped cut sweet bell pepper
- 1 tsp. Herb seasoning blend

Directions:

1. Spread the cheese over the flour wraps. Try to use the ingredients to make two wraps.
2. Layer the tortillas with roast beef, onions, lettuce, pepper strips and cucumber.
3. Sprinkle with the herb seasoning
4. Roll up the wraps and cut them into 4 pieces each. Serve fresh. Enjoy!

Nutrition:

Calories: 255

Protein: 24 g   Sodium: 275 mg

Potassium: 445 mg Phosphorus: 250 mg

CHAPTER 6:

Dinner

71. Crazy Lamb Salad

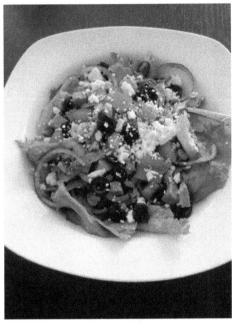

Preparation time: 10 minutes

Cooking Time: 35 minutes

Servings: 4

Ingredients:

- 1 tablespoon olive oil
- 3-pound leg of lamb, bone removed, leg butterflied
- Salt and pepper to taste
- 1 teaspoon cumin
- Pinch of dried thyme
- 2 garlic cloves, peeled and minced

For Salad:

- 4 ounces feta cheese, crumbled
- ½ cup pecans
- 2 cups spinach

- 1 ½ tablespoons lemon juice
- ¼ cup olive oil
- 1 cup fresh mint, chopped

Directions:

1. Rub lamb with salt and pepper, 1 tablespoon oil, thyme, cumin, minced garlic.
2. Pre-heat your grill to medium-high and transfer lamb.
3. Cook for 40 minutes, making sure to flip it once.
4. Take a lined baking sheet and spread the pecans.
5. Toast in oven for 10 minutes at 350-degree F.
6. Transfer grilled lamb to cutting board and let it cool.
7. Slice.
8. Take a salad bowl and add spinach, 1 cup mint, feta cheese, ¼ cup olive oil, lemon juice, toasted pecans, salt, pepper and toss well.
9. Add lamb slices on top.

Nutrition:

Calories: 334

Fat: 33g

Carbohydrates: 5g

Protein: 7g

Phosphorus: 196mg

Potassium: 285mg

Sodium: 111mg

72. Hearty Roasted Cauliflower

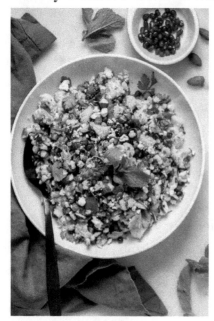

Preparation time: 5 minutes

Cooking Time: 30 minutes

Servings: 8

Ingredients:

- 1 large cauliflower head
- 2 tablespoons melted coconut oil
- 2 tablespoons fresh thyme
- 1 teaspoon Celtic sea sunflower seeds
- 1 teaspoon fresh ground pepper
- 1 head roasted garlic
- 2 tablespoons fresh thyme for garnish

Directions:

1. Pre-heat your oven to 425 degrees F.
2. Rinse cauliflower and trim, core and sliced.
3. Lay cauliflower evenly on rimmed baking tray.
4. Drizzle coconut oil evenly over cauliflower, sprinkle thyme leaves .

5. Season with pinch of sunflower seeds and pepper.
6. Squeeze roasted garlic.
7. Roast cauliflower until slightly caramelized for about 30 minutes, making sure to turn once.
8. Garnish with fresh thyme leaves.
9. Enjoy!

Nutrition:

Calories: 129

Fat: 11g

Carbohydrates: 6g

Protein: 7g

Phosphorus: 296mg

Potassium: 285mg

Sodium: 111mg

73. Cool Cabbage Fried Beef

Preparation time: 5 minutes

Cooking Time: 15 minutes

Servings: 4

Ingredients:

- 1-pound beef, ground and lean
- ½ pound bacon
- 1 onion
- 1 garlic clove, minced
- ½ head cabbage
- Pepper to taste

Directions:

1. Take skillet and place it over medium heat.
2. Add chopped bacon, beef and onion until slightly browned.
3. Transfer to a bowl and keep it covered.
4. Add minced garlic and cabbage to the skillet and cook until slightly browned.

5. Return the ground beef mix to the skillet and simmer for 3-5 minutes over low heat.

6. Serve and enjoy!

Nutrition:

Calories: 360

Fat: 22g

Net Carbohydrates: 5g

Protein: 34g

Phosphorus: 196mg

Potassium: 295mg

Sodium: 121mg

74. Fennel and Figs Lamb

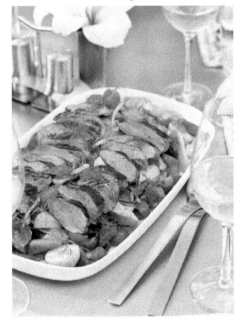

Preparation time: 10 minutes

Cooking Time: 40 minutes

Servings: 2

Ingredients:

- 6 ounces lamb racks
- 1 fennel bulbs, sliced
- pepper to taste
- 1 tablespoon olive oil
- 2 figs, cut in half

- 1/8 cup apple cider vinegar
- 1/2 tablespoon swerve

Directions:

1. Take a bowl and add fennel, figs, vinegar, swerve, oil and toss.

2. Transfer to baking dish.

3. Season with sunflower seeds and pepper.

4. Bake for 15 minutes at 400 degrees F.

5. Season lamb with sunflower seeds and pepper and transfer to a heated pan over medium-high heat.

6. Cook for a few minutes.

7. Add lamb to the baking dish with fennel and bake for 20 minutes.

8. Divide between plates and serve.

9. Enjoy!

Nutrition:

Calories: 230

Fat: 3g

Carbohydrates: 5g

Protein: 10g

Phosphorus: 296mg

Potassium: 225mg

Sodium: 131mg

75. Mushroom and Olive "Mediterranean" Steak

Preparation time: 10 minutes

Cooking Time: 14 minutes

Servings: 2

Ingredients:

- 1/2-pound boneless beef sirloin steak, ¾ inch thick, cut into 4 pieces
- 1/2 large red onion, chopped
- 1/2 cup mushrooms
- 2 garlic cloves, thinly sliced

- 2 tablespoons olive oil
- 1/4 cup green olives, coarsely chopped
- 1/2 cup parsley leaves, finely cut

Directions:

1. Take a large sized skillet and place it over medium-high heat.
2. Add oil and let it heat up.
3. Add beef and cook until both sides are browned, remove beef and drain fat.
4. Add the rest of the oil to the skillet and heat.
5. Add onions, garlic and cook for 2-3 minutes.
6. Stir well.
7. Add mushrooms, olives and cook until the mushrooms are thoroughly done.
8. Return the beef to the skillet and reduce heat to medium.
9. Cook for 3-4 minutes (covered).
10. Stir in parsley.
11. Serve and enjoy!

Nutrition:

Calories: 386 Fat: 30g Carbohydrates: 11g

Protein: 21g Phosphorus: 296mg

Potassium: 295mg Sodium: 111mg

76. Hearty Chicken Fried Rice

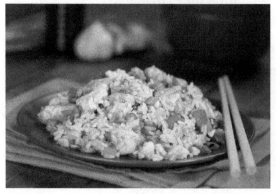

Preparation time: 10 minutes

Cooking Time: 12 minutes

Servings: 4

Ingredients:

- 1 teaspoon olive oil
- 4 large egg whites
- 1 onion, chopped
- 2 garlic cloves, minced
- 12 ounces skinless chicken breasts, boneless, cut into ½ inch cubes
- ½ cup carrots, chopped
- ½ cup frozen green peas
- 2 cups long grain brown rice, cooked
- 3 tablespoons soy sauce, low sodium

Directions:

1. Coat skillet with oil, place it over medium-high heat.
2. Add egg whites and cook until scrambled.
3. Sauté onion, garlic and chicken breasts for 6 minutes.
4. Add carrots, peas and keep cooking for 3 minutes.
5. Stir in rice, season with soy sauce.
6. Add cooked egg whites, stir for 3 minutes.
7. Enjoy!

Nutrition:

Calories: 353

Fat: 11g

Carbohydrates: 30g

Protein: 23g

Phosphorus: 276mg

Potassium: 295mg

Sodium: 134mg

77. Decent Beef and Onion Stew

Preparation time: 10 minutes

Cook Time 1-2 hours

Servings: 4

Ingredients:

- 2 pounds lean beef, cubed
- 3 pounds shallots, peeled
- 5 garlic cloves, peeled, whole
- 3 tablespoons tomato paste
- 1 bay leaves
- ¼ cup olive oil
- 3 tablespoons lemon juice

Directions:

1. Take a stew pot and place it over medium heat.
2. Add olive oil and let it heat up.
3. Add meat and brown.
4. Add remaining ingredients and cover with water.
5. Bring the whole mix to a boil.
6. Reduce heat to low and cover the pot.
7. Simmer for 1-2 hours until beef is cooked thoroughly.
8. Serve hot!

Nutrition:

Calories: 136

Fat: 3g

Carbohydrates: 0.9g

Protein: 24g

Phosphorus: 396mg

Potassium: 205mg

Sodium: 141mg

78. Clean Parsley and Chicken Breast

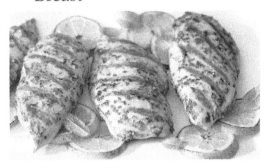

Preparation time: 10 minutes

Cooking Time: 40 minutes

Servings: 2

Ingredients:

- 1/2 tablespoon dry parsley
- 1/2 tablespoon dry basil
- 2 chicken breast halves, boneless and skinless
- 1/4 teaspoon sunflower seeds
- 1/4 teaspoon red pepper flakes, crushed
- 1 tomato, sliced

Directions:

1. Pre-heat your oven to 350 degrees F.
2. Take a 9x13 inch baking dish and grease it up with cooking spray.
3. Sprinkle 1 tablespoon of parsley, 1 teaspoon of basil and spread the mixture over your baking dish.
4. Arrange the chicken breast halves over the dish and sprinkle garlic slices on top.
5. Take a small bowl and add 1 teaspoon parsley, 1 teaspoon of basil, sunflower seeds, basil, red pepper and mix well. Pour the mixture over the chicken breast.
6. Top with tomato slices and cover, bake for 25 minutes.

7. Remove the cover and bake for 15 minutes more.

8. Serve and enjoy!

Nutrition:

Calories: 150 Fat: 4g Carbohydrates: 4g

Protein: 25g Phosphorus: 196mg

Potassium: 285mg Sodium: 111mg

79. Zucchini Beef Sauté with Coriander Greens

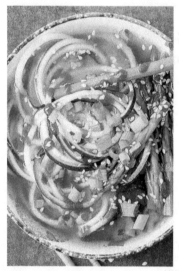

Servings: 4

Preparation time: 10 minutes

Cooking Time: 10 minutes

Ingredients:

- 10 ounces beef, sliced into 1-2-inch strips
- 1 zucchini, cut into 2-inch strips
- ¼ cup parsley, chopped
- 3 garlic cloves, minced
- 2 tablespoons tamari sauce
- 2 tablespoons oil olive

Directions:

1. Add 2 tablespoons olive oil in a frying pan over high heat.

2. Place strips of beef and brown for a few minutes on high heat.

3. Once the meat is brown, add zucchini strips and sauté until tender.

4. Once tender, add tamari sauce, garlic, parsley and let them sit for a few minutes more.

5. Serve immediately and enjoy!

Nutrition:

Calories: 500 Fat: 40g Carbohydrates: 5g

Protein: 31g Phosphorus: 236mg

Potassium: 249mg Sodium: 143mg

80. Hearty Lemon and Pepper Chicken

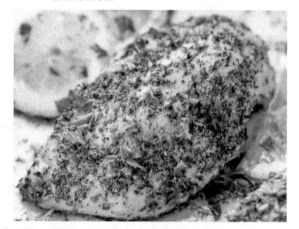

Servings: 4

Preparation time: 5 minutes

Cooking Time: 15

Ingredients:

- 2 teaspoons olive oil
- 1 ¼ pounds skinless chicken cutlets
- 2 whole eggs
- ¼ cup panko crumbs
- 1 tablespoon lemon pepper
- Sunflower seeds and pepper to taste
- 3 cups green beans
- ¼ cup parmesan cheese
- ¼ teaspoon garlic powder

Directions:

1. Pre-heat your oven to 425 degrees F.
2. Take a bowl and stir in seasoning, parmesan, lemon pepper, garlic powder, panko.
3. Whisk eggs in another bowl.
4. Coat cutlets in eggs and press into panko mix.
5. Transfer coated chicken to a parchment lined baking sheet.
6. Toss the beans in oil, pepper, add sunflower seeds, and lay them on the side of the baking sheet.
7. Bake for 15 minutes.
8. Enjoy!

Nutrition:

Calorie: 299

Fat: 10g

Carbohydrates: 10g

Protein: 43g

Phosphorus: 196mg

Potassium: 285mg

Sodium: 111mg

81. Walnuts and Asparagus Delight

Servings: 4

Preparation time: 5 minutes

Cooking Time: 5 minutes

Ingredients:

- 1 ½ tablespoons olive oil
- ¾ pound asparagus, trimmed
- ¼ cup walnuts, chopped
- Sunflower seeds and pepper to taste

Directions:

1. Place a skillet over medium heat add olive oil and let it heat up.
2. Add asparagus, sauté for 5 minutes until browned.
3. Season with sunflower seeds and pepper.
4. Remove heat.
5. Add walnuts and toss.
6. Serve warm!

Nutrition:

Calories: 124 Fat: 12g

Carbohydrates: 2g Protein: 3g

Phosphorus: 196mg Potassium: 205mg

Sodium: 121mg

82. Healthy Carrot Chips

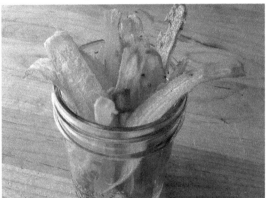

Servings: 4

Preparation time: 10 minutes

Cooking Time: 10 minutes

Ingredients:

- 3 cups carrots, sliced paper-thin rounds
- 2 tablespoons olive oil
- 2 teaspoons ground cumin
- ½ teaspoon smoked paprika
- Pinch of sunflower seeds

Directions:

1. Pre-heat your oven to 400 degrees F.
2. Slice carrot into paper thin shaped coins using a peeler.

3. Place slices in a bowl and toss with oil and spices.

4. Lay out the slices on a parchment paper, lined baking sheet in a single layer.

5. Sprinkle sunflower seeds.

6. Transfer to oven and bake for 8-10 minutes.

7. Remove and serve.

8. Enjoy!

Nutrition:

Calories: 434

Fat: 35g

Carbohydrates: 31g

Protein: 2g

Phosphorus: 196mg

Potassium: 285mg

Sodium: 111mg

Directions:

1. Take a stockpot and add all the ingredients the except heavy cream, salt, and black pepper.

2. Bring to a boil.

3. Reduce heat to simmer.

4. Cook for 40 minutes.

5. Once cooked, warm the heavy cream.

6. Then add once the soup is cooked.

7. Blend the soup till smooth by using an immersion blender.

8. Season with salt and black pepper.

9. Serve and enjoy!

Nutrition:

Calories: 270 Fat: 14g

Carbohydrates: 6g Protein: 29g

Phosphorus: 187mg Potassium: 258mg

Sodium: 145mg

83. Beef Soup

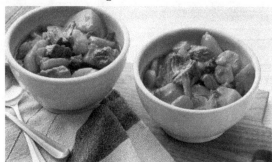

Servings: 4

Preparation time: 10 minutes

Cooking Time: 40 minutes

Ingredients:

- 1-pound ground beef, lean
- 1 cup mixed vegetables, frozen
- 1 yellow onion,chopped
- 6 cups vegetable broth
- 1 cup low-fat cream
- Pepper to taste

84. Amazing Grilled Chicken and Blueberry Salad

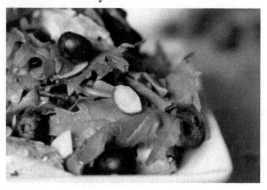

Servings: 5

Preparation time: 10 minutes

Cooking Time: 25 minutes

Ingredients:

- 5 cups mixed greens
- 1 cup blueberries
- ¼ cup slivered almonds

- 2 cups chicken breasts, cooked and cubed

For dressing:

- ¼ cup olive oil
- ¼ cup apple cider vinegar
- ¼ cup blueberries
- 2 tablespoons honey
- Sunflower seeds and pepper to taste

Directions:

1. Take a bowl and add greens, berries, almonds, chicken cubes and mix well.
2. Take a bowl and mix the dressing ingredients, pour the mix into a blender and blitz until smooth.
3. Add dressing on top of the chicken cubes and toss well.
4. Season more and enjoy!

Nutrition:

Calories: 266 Fat: 17g

Carbohydrates: 18g Protein: 10g

Phosphorus: 196mg Potassium: 285mg

Sodium: 91mg

85. Clean Chicken and Mushroom Stew

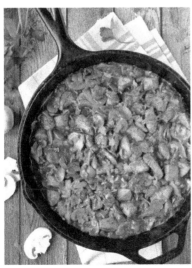

Servings: 4

Preparation time: 10 minutes

Cooking Time: 35 minutes

Ingredients:

- 4 chicken breast halves, cut into bite sized pieces
- 1-pound mushrooms, sliced (5-6 cups)
- 1 bunch spring onion, chopped
- 4 tablespoons olive oil
- 1 teaspoon thyme
- Sunflower seeds and pepper as needed

Directions:

1. Take a large deep-frying pan and place it over medium-high heat.
2. Add oil and let it heat up.
3. Add chicken and cook for 4-5 minutes per side until slightly browned.
4. Add spring onions and mushrooms, season with sunflower seeds and pepper according to your taste.
5. Stir.
6. Cover with lid and bring the mix to a boil.
7. Reduce heat and simmer for 25 minutes.
8. Serve!

Nutrition:

Calories: 247

Fat: 12g

Carbohydrates: 10g

Protein: 23g

Phosphorus: 296mg

Potassium: 215mg

Sodium: 87mg

86. Elegant Pumpkin Chili Dish

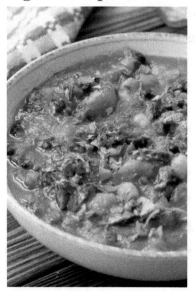

Servings: 4

Preparation time: 10 minutes

Cooking Time: 15 minutes

Ingredients:

- 3 cups yellow onion, chopped
- 8 garlic cloves, chopped
- 1-pound turkey, ground
- 2 cans (15 ounces each) fire roasted tomatoes
- 2 cups pumpkin puree
- 1 cup chicken broth
- 4 teaspoons chili spice
- 1 teaspoon ground cinnamon
- 1 teaspoon sea sunflower seeds

Directions:

1. Take a large sized pot and place it over medium-high heat.
2. Add coconut oil and let the oil heat up.
3. Add onion and garlic, sauté for 5 minutes.
4. Add ground turkey and break it while cooking, cook for 5 minutes.

5. Add remaining ingredients and bring the mix to simmer.
6. Simmer for 15 minutes over low heat (lid off).
7. Pour chicken broth.
8. Serve with desired salad.
9. Enjoy!

Nutrition:

Calories: 312 Fat: 16g Carbohydrates: 14g

Protein: 27g Phosphorus: 196mg

Potassium: 285mg Sodium: 171mg

87. Zucchini Zoodles with Chicken and Basil

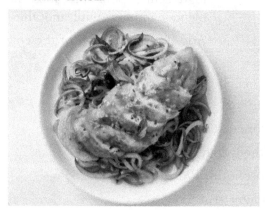

Servings: 2

Preparation time: 10 minutes

Cooking Time: 10 minutes

Ingredients:

- 2 chicken fillets, cubed
- 2 tablespoons ghee
- 1-pound tomatoes, diced
- ½ cup basil, chopped
- ¼ cup coconut almond milk
- 1 garlic clove, peeled, minced
- 1 zucchini, shredded

Directions:

1. Sauté cubed chicken in ghee until no longer pink.

2. Add tomatoes and season with sunflower seeds.

3. Simmer and reduce the liquid.

4. Prepare your zucchini Zoodles by shredding zucchini in a food processor.

5. Add basil, garlic, coconut almond milk to chicken and cook for a few minutes.

6. Add half of the zucchini Zoodles to a bowl and top with creamy tomato basil chicken.

7. Enjoy!

Nutrition:

Calories: 540 Fat: 27g

Carbohydrates: 13g Protein: 59g

Phosphorus: 236mg Potassium: 290mg

Sodium: 128mg

88. Tasty Roasted Broccoli

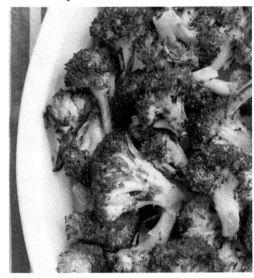

Servings: 4

Preparation time: 5 minutes

Cooking Time: 20 minutes

Ingredients:

- 4 cups broccoli florets
- 1 tablespoon olive oil

- Sunflower seeds and pepper to taste

Directions:

1. Pre-heat your oven to 400 degrees F.

2. Add broccoli in a zip bag alongside oil and shake until coated.

3. Add seasoning and shake again.

4. Spread broccoli out on baking sheet, bake for 20 minutes.

5. Let it cool and serve.

6. Enjoy!

Nutrition:

Calories: 62

Fat: 4g

Carbohydrates: 4g

Protein: 4g

Phosphorus: 267mg

Potassium: 285mg

Sodium: 134mg

89. The Almond Breaded Chicken Goodness

Servings: 3

Preparation time: 15 minutes

Cooking Time: 15 minutes

Ingredients:

- 2 large chicken breasts, boneless and skinless
- 1/3 cup lemon juice
- 1 ½ cups seasoned almond meal
- 2 tablespoons coconut oil
- Lemon pepper, to taste
- Parsley for decoration

Directions:

1. Slice chicken breast in half.

2. Pound out each half until ¼ inch thick.

3. Take a pan and place it over medium heat, add oil and heat it.

4. Dip each chicken breast slice into lemon juice and let it sit for 2 minutes.

5. Turnover and the let the other side sit for 2 minutes as well.

6. Transfer to almond meal and coat both sides.

7. Add coated chicken to the oil and fry for 4 minutes per side, making sure to sprinkle lemon pepper liberally.

8. Transfer to a paper lined sheet and repeat until all chicken are fried.

9. Garnish with parsley and enjoy!

Nutrition:

Calories: 325 Fat: 24g Carbohydrates: 3g

Protein: 16g Phosphorus: 196mg

Potassium: 285mg Sodium: 111mg

90. South-Western Pork Chops

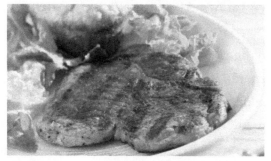

Servings: 4

Preparation time: 10 minutes

Cooking Time: 15 minutes

Ingredients:

- Cooking spray as needed
- 4-ounce pork loin chop, boneless and fat rimmed
- 1/3 cup salsa
- 2 tablespoons fresh lime juice
- ¼ cup fresh cilantro, chopped

Directions:

1. Take a large sized non-stick skillet and spray it with cooking spray.

2. Heat until hot over high heat.

3. Press the chops with your palm to flatten them slightly.

4. Add them to the skillet and cook on 1 minute for each side until they are nicely browned.

5. Lower the heat to medium-low.

6. Combine the salsa and lime juice.

7. Pour the mix over the chops.

8. Simmer uncovered for about 8 minutes until the chops are perfectly done.

9. If needed, sprinkle some cilantro on top.

Nutrition:

Calorie: 184 Fat: 4g Carbohydrates: 4g

Protein: 0.5g Phosphorus: 196mg

Potassium: 285mg Sodium: 98mg

91. Almond butter Pork Chops

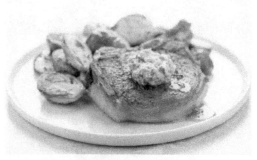

Servings: 2

Preparation time: 5 minutes

Cooking Time: 25 minutes

Ingredients:

- 1 tablespoon almond butter, divided
- 2 boneless pork chops
- Pepper to taste

- 1 tablespoon dried Italian seasoning, low fat and low sodium
- 1 tablespoon olive oil

Directions:

1. Pre-heat your oven to 350 degrees F.
2. Pat pork chops dry with a paper towel and place them in a baking dish.
3. Season with pepper, and Italian seasoning.
4. Drizzle olive oil over pork chops.
5. Top each chop with ½ tablespoon almond butter.
6. Bake for 25 minutes.
7. Transfer pork chops on two plates and top with almond butter juice.
8. Serve and enjoy!

Nutrition:

Calories: 333

Fat: 23g

Carbohydrates: 1g

Protein: 31g

Phosphorus: 296mg

Potassium: 285mg

Sodium: 123mg

92. Chicken Salsa

Servings: 1

Preparation time: 4 minutes

Cooking Time: 14 minutes

Ingredients:

- 2 chicken breasts
- 1 cup salsa
- 1 taco seasoning mix
- 1 cup plain Greek Yogurt
- ½ cup of kite ricotta/cashew cheese, cubed

Directions:

1. Take a skillet and place over medium heat.
2. Add chicken breast, ½ cup of salsa and taco seasoning.
3. Mix well and cook for 12-15 minutes until the chicken is done.
4. Take the chicken out and cube them.
5. Place the cubes on toothpick and top with cheddar.
6. Place yogurt and remaining salsa in cups and use as dips.
7. Enjoy!

Nutrition:

Calories: 359 Fat: 14g

Net Carbohydrates: 14g Protein: 43g

Phosphorus: 196mg Potassium: 285mg

Sodium: 111mg

93. Healthy Mediterranean Lamb Chops

Servings: 4

Preparation time: 10 minutes

Cooking Time: 10 minutes

Ingredients:

- 4 lamb shoulder chops, 8 ounces each
- 2 tablespoons Dijon mustard
- 2 tablespoons Balsamic vinegar
- ½ cup olive oil
- 2 tablespoons shredded fresh basil

Directions:

1. Pat your lamb chop dry using a kitchen towel and arrange them on a shallow glass baking dish.

2. Take a bowl and a whisk in Dijon mustard, balsamic vinegar, pepper and mix them well.

3. Whisk in the oil very slowly into the marinade until the mixture is smooth

4. Stir in basil.

5. Pour the marinade over the lamb chops and stir to coat both sides well.

6. Cover the chops and allow them to marinate for 1-4 hours (chilled).

7. Take the chops out and leave them for 30 minutes to allow the temperature to reach an average level.

8. Pre-heat your grill to medium heat and add oil to the grate.

9. Grill the lamb chops for 5-10 minutes per side until both sides are browned.

10. Once the center reads 145 degrees F, the chops are ready, serve and enjoy!

Nutrition:

Calories: 521 Fat: 45g

Carbohydrates: 3.5g

Protein: 22g

Phosphorus: 226mg

Potassium: 295mg

Sodium: 111mg

94. Amazing Sesame Breadsticks

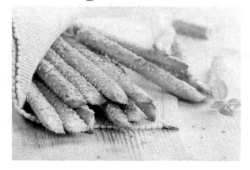

Servings: 5 breadsticks

Preparation time: 10 minutes

Cooking Time: 20 minutes

Ingredients:

- 1 egg white
- 2 tablespoons almond flour
- 1 teaspoon Himalayan pink sunflower seeds
- 1 tablespoon extra-virgin olive oil
- ½ teaspoon sesame seeds

Directions:

1. Pre-heat your oven to 320 degrees F.

2. Line a baking sheet with parchment paper and keep it on the side.

3. Take a bowl and whisk in egg whites, add flour and half of sunflower seeds and olive oil.

4. Knead until you have a smooth dough.

5. Divide into 4 pieces and roll into breadsticks.

6. Place on prepared sheet and brush with olive oil, sprinkle sesame seeds and remaining sunflower seeds.

7. Bake for 20 minutes.

8. Serve and enjoy!

Nutrition:

Total Carbs: 1.1g

Fiber: 1g

Protein: 1.6g

Fat: 5g

Phosphorus: 196mg

Potassium: 285mg

Sodium: 111mg

95. Brown Butter Duck Breast

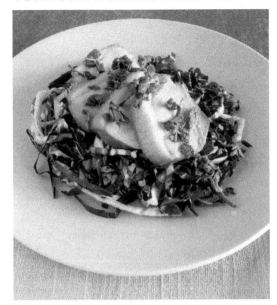

Servings: 3

Preparation time: 5 minutes

Cooking Time: 25 minutes

Ingredients:

- 1 whole 6-ounce duck breast, skin on
- Pepper to taste
- 1 head radicchio, 4 ounces, core removed
- ¼ cup unsalted butter
- 6 fresh sage leaves, sliced

Directions:

1. Pre-heat your oven to 400-degree F.
2. Pat duck breast dry with paper towel.
3. Season with pepper.
4. Place duck breast in skillet and place it over medium heat, sear for 3-4 minutes each side.
5. Turn breast over and transfer skillet to oven.
6. Roast for 10 minutes (uncovered).
7. Cut radicchio in half.
8. Remove and discard the woody white core and thinly slice the leaves.
9. Keep them on the side.
10. Remove skillet from oven.
11. Transfer duck breast, fat side up to cutting board and let it rest.
12. Re-heat your skillet over medium heat.
13. Add unsalted butter, sage and cook for 3-4 minutes.
14. Cut duck into 6 equal slices.
15. Divide radicchio between 2 plates, top with slices of duck breast and drizzle browned butter and sage.

Nutrition:

Calories: 393 Fat: 33g

Carbohydrates: 2g

Protein: 22g

Phosphorus: 196mg

Potassium: 285mg

Sodium: 143mg

96. Generous Garlic Bread Stick

Servings: 8 breadsticks

Preparation time: 15 minutes

Cooking Time: 15 minutes

Ingredients:

- ¼ cup almond butter, softened
- 1 teaspoon garlic powder
- 2 cups almond flour
- ½ tablespoon baking powder
- 1 tablespoon Psyllium husk powder
- ¼ teaspoon sunflower seeds
- 3 tablespoons almond butter, melted
- 1 egg
- ¼ cup boiling water

Directions:

1. Pre-heat your oven to 400 degrees F.
2. Line baking sheet with parchment paper and keep it on the side.
3. Beat almond butter with garlic powder and keep it on the side.
4. Add almond flour, baking powder, husk, sunflower seeds in a bowl and mix in almond butter and egg, mix well.
5. Pour boiling water in the mix and stir until you have a nice dough.
6. Divide the dough into 8 balls and roll into breadsticks.
7. Place on baking sheet and bake for 15 minutes.
8. Brush each stick with garlic almond butter and bake for 5 minutes more.
9. Serve and enjoy!

Nutrition:

Total Carbs: 7g Fiber: 2g Protein: 7g

Fat: 24g Phosphorus: 276mg

Potassium: 289mg Sodium: 101mg

97. Cauliflower Bread Stick

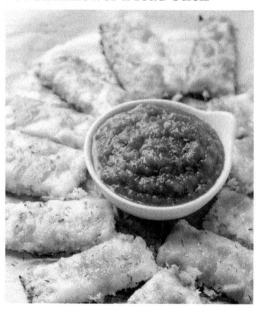

Servings: 5 breadsticks

Preparation time: 10 minutes

Cooking Time: 48 minutes

Ingredients:

- 1 cup cashew cheese/ kite ricotta cheese
- 1 tablespoon organic almond butter
- 1 whole egg
- ½ teaspoon Italian seasoning
- ¼ teaspoon red pepper flakes
- 1/8 teaspoon kosher sunflower seeds
- 2 cups cauliflower rice, cooked for 3 minutes in microwave
- 3 teaspoons garlic, minced
- Parmesan cheese, grated

Directions:

1. Pre-heat your oven to 350 degrees F.
2. Add almond butter in a small pan and melt over low heat
3. Add red pepper flakes, garlic to the almond butter and cook for 2-3 minutes.
4. Add garlic and almond butter mix to the bowl with cooked cauliflower and add the Italian seasoning.
5. Season with sunflower seeds and mix, refrigerate for 10 minutes.
6. Add cheese and eggs to the bowl and mix.
7. Place a layer of parchment paper at the bottom of a 9 x 9 baking dish and grease with cooking spray, add egg and mozzarella cheese mix to the cauliflower mix.
8. Add mix to the pan and smooth to a thin layer with the palms of your hand.

9. Bake for 30 minutes, take out from oven and top with few shakes of parmesan and mozzarella.

10. Cook for 8 minutes more.

Nutrition:

Total Carbs: 11.5g

Fiber: 2g

Protein: 10.7g

Fat: 20g

Phosphorus: 316mg

Potassium: 285mg

Sodium: 87mg

98. Bacon and Chicken Garlic Wrap

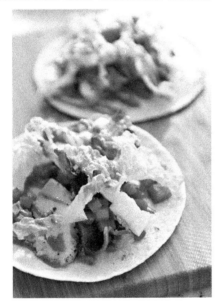

Servings: 4

Preparation time: 15 minutes

Cooking Time: 10 minutes

Ingredients:

- 1 chicken fillet, cut into small cubes
- 8-9 thin slices bacon, cut to fit cubes
- 6 garlic cloves, minced

Directions:

1. Pre-heat your oven to 400 degrees F.

2. Line a baking tray with aluminum foil.

3. Add minced garlic to a bowl and rub each chicken piece with it.

4. Wrap a bacon piece around each garlic chicken bite.

5. Secure with toothpick.

6. Transfer bites to baking sheet, keeping a little bit of space between them.

7. Bake for about 15-20 minutes until crispy.

8. Serve and enjoy!

Nutrition:

Calories: 260 Fat: 19g Carbohydrates: 5g

Protein: 22g Phosphorus: 276mg

Potassium: 285mg Sodium: 121mg

99. Chipotle Lettuce Chicken

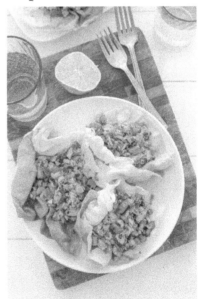

Servings: 6

Preparation time: 10 minutes

Cooking Time: 25 minutes

Ingredients:

- 1-pound chicken breast, cut into strips

- Splash of olive oil
- 1 red onion, finely sliced
- 14 ounces tomatoes
- 1 teaspoon chipotle, chopped
- ½ teaspoon cumin
- Lettuce as needed
- Fresh coriander leaves
- Jalapeno chilies, sliced
- Fresh tomato slices for garnish
- Lime wedges

Directions:

1. Take a non-stick frying pan and place it over medium heat.
2. Add oil and heat it up.
3. Add chicken and cook until brown.
4. Keep the chicken on the side.
5. Add tomatoes, sugar, chipotle, cumin to the same pan and simmer for 25 minutes until you have a nice sauce.
6. Add chicken into the sauce and cook for 5 minutes.
7. Transfer the mix to another place.
8. Use lettuce wraps to take a portion of the mixture and serve with a squeeze of lemon.
9. Enjoy!

Nutrition:

Calories: 332

Fat: 15g

Carbohydrates: 13g

Protein: 34g

Phosphorus: 196mg

Potassium: 285mg

Sodium: 111mg

100.   Eggplant and Red Pepper Soup

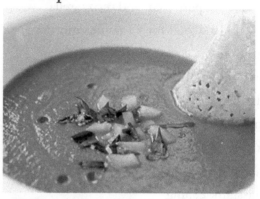

Preparation time: 20 minutes

Cooking Time: 40 minutes

Servings: 6

Ingredients:

- Sweet onion – 1 small, cut into quarters
- Small red bell peppers – 2, halved
- Cubed eggplant – 2 cups
- Garlic – 2 cloves, crushed
- Olive oil – 1 Tablespoon.
- Chicken stock – 1 cup
- Water
- Chopped fresh basil – ¼ cup
- Ground black pepper

Directions:

1. Preheat the oven to 350F.
2. Put the onions, red peppers, eggplant, and garlic in a baking dish.
3. Drizzle the vegetables with the olive oil.
4. Roast the vegetables for 30 minutes or until they are slightly charred and soft.
5. Cool the vegetables slightly and remove the skin from the peppers.
6. Puree the vegetables with a hand mixer (with the chicken stock).

7. Transfer the soup to a medium pot and add enough water to reach the desired thickness.

8. Heat the soup to a simmer and add the basil.

9. Season with pepper and serve.

Nutrition:

Calories: 61

Fat: 2g

Carb: 9g

Phosphorus: 33mg

Potassium: 198mg

Sodium: 98mg

Protein: 2g

101.   Seafood Casserole

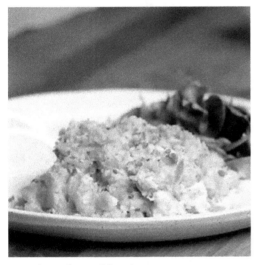

Preparation time: 20 minutes

Cooking Time: 45 minutes

Servings: 6

Ingredients:

- Eggplant – 2 cups, peeled and diced into 1-inch pieces
- Butter, for greasing the baking dish
- Olive oil – 1 tablespoon.
- Sweet onion – ½, chopped
- Minced garlic - 1 teaspoon.
- Celery stalk – 1, chopped
- Red bell pepper – ½, boiled and chopped
- Freshly squeezed lemon juice – 3 Tablespoons.
- Hot sauce – 1 teaspoon.
- Creole seasoning mix – ¼ teaspoon.
- White rice – ½ cup, uncooked
- Egg – 1 large
- Cooked shrimp – 4 ounces
- Queen crab meat – 6 ounces

Directions:

1. Preheat the oven to 350F.

2. Boil the eggplant in a saucepan for 5 minutes. Drain and set aside.

3. Grease a 9-by-13-inch baking dish with butter and set aside.

4. Heat the olive oil in a large skillet over medium heat.

5. Sauté the garlic, onion, celery, and bell pepper for 4 minutes or until tender.

6. Add the sautéed vegetables to the eggplant, along with the lemon juice, hot sauce, seasoning, rice, and egg.

7. Stir to combine.

8. Fold in the shrimp and crab meat.

9. Spoon the casserole mixture into the casserole dish, patting down the top.

10. Bake for 25 to 30 minutes or until casserole is heated through and rice is tender.

11. Serve warm.

Nutrition:

Calories: 118 Fat: 4g

Carb: 9g Phosphorus: 102mg

Potassium: 199mg

Sodium: 235mg Protein: 12g

102. Ground Beef and Rice Soup

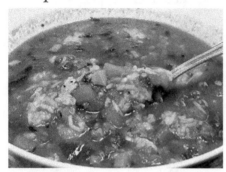

Preparation time: 15 minutes

Cooking Time: 40 minutes

Servings: 6

Ingredients:

- Extra-lean ground beef – ½ pound
- Small sweet onion – ½, chopped
- Minced garlic – 1 teaspoon.
- Water – 2 cups
- Low-sodium beef broth – 1 cup
- Long-grain white rice – ½ cup, uncooked
- Celery stalk – 1, chopped
- Fresh green beans – ½ cup, cut into – 1-inch pieces
- Chopped fresh thyme – 1 teaspoon.
- Ground black pepper

Directions:

1. Sauté the ground beef in a saucepan for 6 minutes or until the beef is completely browned.
2. Drain off the excess fat and add the onion and garlic to the saucepan.
3. Sauté the vegetables for about 3 minutes, or until they are softened.
4. Add the celery, rice, beef broth, and water.
5. Bring the soup to a boil, reduce the heat to low and simmer for 30 minutes or until the rice is tender.

6. Add the green beans and thyme and simmer for 3 minutes.
7. Remove the soup from the heat and season with pepper.

Nutrition:

Calories: 154 Fat: 7g Carb: 14g

Phosphorus: 76mg Potassium: 179mg

Sodium: 133mg Protein: 9g

103. Couscous Burgers

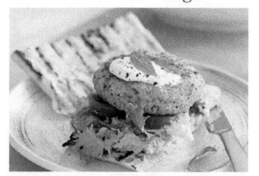

Preparation time: 20 minutes

Cooking Time: 10 minutes

Servings: 6

Ingredients:

- Canned chickpeas – ½ cup, rinsed and drained
- Chopped fresh cilantro – 2 Tablespoons.
- Chopped fresh parsley
- Lemon juice - 1 Tablespoon.
- Lemon zest – 2 teaspoons.
- Minced garlic – 1 teaspoon.
- Cooked couscous – 2 ½ cups
- Eggs – 2 lightly beaten
- Olive oil – 2 Tablespoons.

Directions:

1. Put the cilantro, chickpeas, parsley, lemon juice, lemon zest, and garlic

in a food processor and pulse until a paste forms.

2. Transfer the chickpea mixture to a bowl and add the eggs and couscous. Mix well.

3. Chill the mixture in the refrigerator for 1 hour.

4. Form the couscous mixture into 4 patties.

5. Heat olive oil in a skillet.

6. Place the patties in the skillet, 2 at a time, gently pressing them down with a spatula.

7. Cook for 5 minutes or until golden and flip the patties over.

8. Cook the other side for 5 minutes and transfer the cooked burgers to a plate covered with a paper towel.

9. Repeat with the remaining 2 burgers.

Nutrition:

Calories: 242 Fat: 10g Carb: 29g

Phosphorus: 108mg Potassium: 168mg

Sodium: 43mg Protein: 9g

104.   Baked Flounder

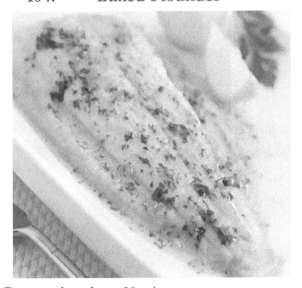

Preparation time: 20 minutes

Cooking Time: 5 minutes

Servings: 4

Ingredients:

- Homemade mayonnaise – ¼ cup
- Juice of 1 lime
- Zest of 1 lime
- Chopped fresh cilantro – ½ cup
- Flounder fillets – 4 (3-ounce)
- Ground black pepper

Directions:

1. Preheat the oven to 400F.

2. In a bowl, stir together the cilantro, lime juice, lime zest, and mayonnaise.

3. Place 4 pieces of foil, about 8 by 8 inches square, on a clean work surface.

4. Place a flounder fillet in the center of each square.

5. Top the fillets evenly with the mayonnaise mixture.

6. Season the flounder with pepper.

7. Fold the foil's sides over the fish, create a snug packet, and place the foil packets on a baking sheet.

8. Bake the fish for 4 to 5 minutes.

9. Unfold the packets and serve.

Nutrition:

Calories: 92

Fat: 4g

Carb: 2g

Phosphorus: 208mg

Potassium: 137mg

Sodium: 267mg

Protein: 12g

105.   Persian Chicken

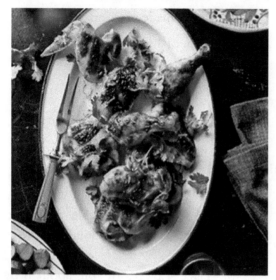

Preparation time: 10 minutes

Cooking Time: 20 minutes

Servings: 5

Ingredients:

- Sweet onion – ½, chopped
- Lemon juice – ¼ cup
- Dried oregano – 1 Tablespoon.
- Minced garlic – 1 teaspoon.
- Sweet paprika – 1 teaspoon.
- Ground cumin – ½ teaspoon.
- Olive oil – ½ cup
- Boneless, skinless chicken thighs – 5

Directions:

1. Put the cumin, paprika, garlic, oregano, lemon juice, and onion in a food processor and pulse to mix the ingredients.
2. Keep the motor running and add the olive oil until the mixture is smooth.
3. Place the chicken thighs in a large sealable freezer bag and pour the marinade into the bag.
4. Seal the bag and place in the refrigerator, turning the bag twice, for 2 hours.
5. Remove the thighs from the marinade and discard the extra marinade.
6. Preheat the barbecue to medium.
7. Grill the chicken for about 20 minutes, turning once, until it reaches 165F.

Nutrition:

Calories: 321

Fat: 21g

Carb: 3g

Phosphorus: 131mg

Potassium: 220mg

Sodium: 86mg

Protein: 22g

106.   Pork Souvlaki

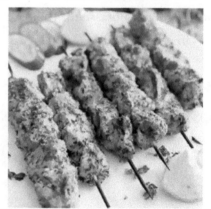

Preparation time: 20 minutes

Cooking Time: 12 minutes

Servings: 8

Ingredients:

- Olive oil – 3 Tablespoons.
- Lemon juice – 2 Tablespoons.
- Minced garlic – 1 teaspoon.
- Chopped fresh oregano – 1 Tablespoon.

- Ground black pepper – ¼ teaspoon.
- Pork leg – 1 pound, cut in 2-inch cubes

Directions:

1. In a bowl, stir together the lemon juice, olive oil, garlic, oregano, and pepper.
2. Add the pork cubes and toss to coat.
3. Place the bowl in the refrigerator, covered, for 2 hours to marinate.
4. Thread the pork chunks onto 8 wooden skewers that have been soaked in water.
5. Preheat the barbecue to medium-high heat.
6. Grill the pork skewers for about 12 minutes, turning once, until just cooked through but still juicy.

Nutrition:

Calories: 95 Fat: 4g Carb: 0g

Phosphorus: 125mg

Potassium: 230mg Sodium: 29mg Protein: 13g

107.   Pork Meatloaf

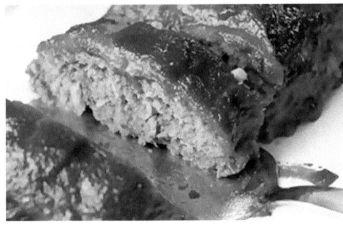

Preparation time: 10 minutes

Cooking Time: 50 minutes

Servings: 8

Ingredients:

- 95% lean ground beef – 1 pound

- Breadcrumbs – ½ cup
- Chopped sweet onion – ½ cup
- Egg – 1
- Chopped fresh basil – 2 Tablespoons.
- Chopped fresh thyme -1 teaspoon.
- Chopped fresh parsley – 1 teaspoon.
- Ground black pepper – ¼ teaspoon.
- Brown sugar – 1 Tablespoon.
- White vinegar – 1 teaspoon.
- Garlic powder – ¼ teaspoon.

Directions:

1. Preheat the oven to 350F.
2. Mix together the breadcrumbs, beef, onion, basil, egg, thyme, parsley, and pepper until well combined.
3. Press the meat mixture into a 9-by-5-inch loaf pan.
4. In a small bowl, stir together the brown sugar, vinegar, and garlic powder.
5. Spread the brown sugar mixture evenly over the meat.
6. Bake the meatloaf for about 50 minutes or until it is cooked through.
7. Let the meatloaf stand for 10 minutes and then pour out any accumulated grease.

Nutrition:

Calories: 103 Fat: 3g

Carb: 7g Phosphorus: 112mg

Potassium: 190mg

Sodium: 87mg

Protein: 11g

108.   Chicken Stew

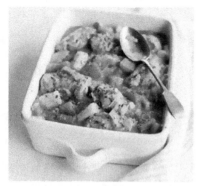

Preparation time: 20 minutes

Cooking Time: 50 minutes

Servings: 6

Ingredients:

- Olive oil – 1 Tablespoon.
- Boneless, skinless chicken thighs – 1 pound, cut into 1-inch cubes
- Sweet onion – ½, chopped
- Minced garlic – 1 Tablespoon.
- Chicken stock – 2 cups
- Water – 1 cup, plus 2 Tablespoons.
- Carrot – 1, sliced
- Celery – 2 stalks, sliced
- Turnip – 1, sliced thin
- Chopped fresh thyme – 1 Tablespoon.
- Chopped fresh rosemary – 1 teaspoon.
- Cornstarch – 2 teaspoons.
- Ground black pepper to taste

Directions:

1. Place a large saucepan on medium heat and add the olive oil.
2. Sauté the chicken for 6 minutes or until it is lightly browned, stirring often.
3. Add the onion and garlic, and sauté for 3 minutes.
4. Add 1-cup water, chicken stock, carrot, celery, and turnip and bring the stew to a boil.
5. Reduce the heat to low and simmer for 30 minutes or until the chicken is cooked through and tender.
6. Add the thyme and rosemary and simmer for 3 minutes more.
7. In a small bowl, stir together the 2 tablespoons. Of water and the cornstarch; add the mixture to the stew.
8. Stir to incorporate the cornstarch mixture and cook for 3 to 4 minutes or until the stew thickens.
9. Remove from the heat and season with pepper.

Nutrition:

Calories: 141 Fat: 8g Carb: 5g

Phosphorus: 53mg Potassium: 192mg

Sodium: 214mg Protein: 9g

109.   Beef Chili

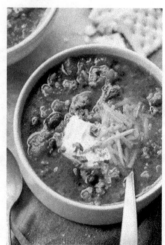

Preparation time: 10 minutes

Cooking Time: 30 minutes

Servings: 2

Ingredients:

- Onion – 1, diced

- Red bell pepper – 1, diced
- Garlic – 2 cloves, minced
- Lean ground beef – 6 oz.
- Chili powder – 1 teaspoon.
- Oregano – 1 teaspoon.
- Extra virgin olive oil – 2 Tablespoons.
- Water – 1 cup
- Brown rice -1 cup
- Fresh cilantro – 1 Tablespoon. to serve

Directions:

1. Soak vegetables in warm water.
2. Bring a pan of water to the boil and add rice for 20 minutes.
3. Meanwhile, add the oil to a pan and heat on medium-high heat.
4. Add the pepper, onions, and garlic and sauté for 5 minutes until soft.
5. Remove and set aside.
6. Add the beef to the pan and stir until browned.
7. Add the vegetables back into the pan and stir.
8. Now add the chili powder and herbs and the water, cover and turn the heat down a little to simmer for 15 minutes.
9. Meanwhile, drain the water from the rice, and the lid and steam while the chili is cooking.
10. Serve hot with the fresh cilantro sprinkled over the top.

Nutrition:

Calories: 459 Fat: 22g

Carb: 36g Phosphorus: 332mg

Potassium: 360mg Sodium: 33mg

Protein: 22g

Crab Cakes

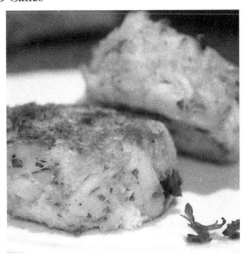

Preparation Time: 10 minutes

Cooking Time: 20 minutes

Servings: 4

Ingredients:

- 1 lb. crab meat
- 1 egg
- 1/3 cup bell pepper, chopped
- 1/4 cup onion, chopped
- 1/4 cup panko breadcrumbs
- 1/4 cup mayonnaise
- 1 tablespoon dry mustard
- 1 teaspoon black pepper
- 2 tablespoons lemon juice
- 1 tablespoon garlic powder
- Dash cayenne pepper
- 3 tablespoons olive oil

Direction:

1. Mix the crab meat with all the spices, veggies, crackers, egg, and mayonnaise in a suitable bowl.
2. Once it is well mixed, make 4 patties out of this mixture.
3. Grease a suitable skillet and place it over moderate heat.

4. Sear each Pattie for 5 minutes per side in the hot pan.

5. Serve.

Nutrition:

Calories 315Total Fat 20.4g

Saturated Fat 2.9g Cholesterol 105mg

Sodium 844mg Protein 17.4g Calcium 437mg

Phosphorous 288mg Potassium 114mg

110.   Fried   Wine   Octopus Patties

Preparation Time: 10 minutes

Cooking Time: 10 minutes

Servings: 6

Ingredients:

- 2 lbs. octopus fresh or frozen, cleaned and cut in small cubes
- 1 cup of ground almond
- 1 cup of red wine
- 2 spring onions finely chopped
- 1 Tablespoon of oregano
- Salt and ground black pepper
- 1 cup of olive oil

Directions:

1. In a deep bowl, combine the octopus cubes, ground almond, red wine, spring onions, oregano, salt, and pepper.

2. Knead until combined well.

3. Form the mixture into balls or patties.

4. Heat the oil in a large and deep fry pan.

5. Fry octopus patties until get a golden color.

6. Transfer the octopus patties on a platter lined with kitchen paper towel. Serve warm.

Nutrition:

Calories: 526 Carbohydrates: 8g

Proteins: 28g Fat: 49.5g Fiber: 3g

111.   Grilled King Prawns with Parsley Sauce

Preparation Time: 10 minutes

Cooking Time: 15 minutes

Servings: 4

Ingredients:

- 40 king prawns, heads off and unpeeled
- 1/4 cup olive oil
- 2 green onions (scallions), finely chopped
- 2 Tbsp of fresh parsley, finely chopped
- 3 Tbsp water
- Salt and pepper to taste

Directions:

1. Cut prawns in half so that the meat is exposed in the shell.

2. In a large skillet heat the olive oil and sauté the green onion for 2 - 3 minutes or until softened.

3. Add chopped parsley, water, salt and pepper: stir for 2 minutes and remove from the heat.

4. Preheat your grill (pellet, gas, charcoal) to HIGH according to manufacturer Instructions.

5. Brush prawns with onion - parsley mixture, and grill for 3 - 4 each side.

6.   Serve hot.

Nutrition:

Calories: 209

Carbohydrates: 3g

Proteins: 38g

Fat: 4g

Fiber: 0.3g

112. Cajun Lime Grilled Shrimp

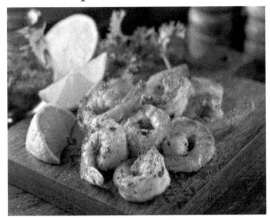

Preparation Time: 10 minutes

Cooking Time: 15 minutes

Servings: 6

Ingredients:

- 3 Tbsp Cajun seasoning
- 2 lime, juiced
- 2 Tbsp olive oil
- 1 lbs. peeled and deveined medium shrimp (30-40 per pound)

Directions:

1. Mix together the Cajun seasoning, lime juice, and olive oil in a resalable plastic bag.
2. Add the shrimp, coat with the marinade, squeeze out excess air, and seal the bag.
3. Marinate in the refrigerator for 20 minutes.
4. Preheat your grill (pellet, gas, charcoal) to HIGH according to manufacturer Instructions.
5. Remove the shrimp from the marinade and shake off excess. Discard the remaining marinade.
6. Grill shrimp until they are bright pink on the outside and the meat is no longer transparent in the center, about 2 minutes per side.
7. Serve hot.

Nutrition:

Calories: 318

Carbohydrates: 8.7g

Proteins: 32g

Fat: 17g

Fiber: 3g

113. Iberian Shrimp Fritters

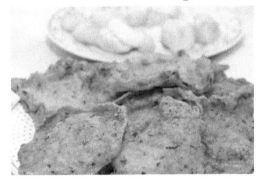

Preparation Time: 10 minutes

Cooking Time: 5 minutes

Servings: 4

Ingredients:

- 1 green onion, finely diced
- 1 lbs. raw shrimp, peeled, deveined, and finely chopped
- 1 cup almond flour
- 2 Tbsp fresh parsley (chopped)
- 1 tsp baking powder
- 1 tsp hot paprika
- Salt and freshly ground black pepper, to taste
- 1/4 cup olive oil
- Lemon wedges, for serving

Directions:

1. In a broad and deep bowl, combine green onions, shrimp, almond flour, parsley, baking powder, paprika, and pinch of the salt and pepper.
2. Form mixture in patties/balls/fritters.

3. Heat the oil in a large skillet over high heat.

4. Fry shrimp fritters for about 5 minutes in total turning once or twice.

5. Using a spatula, transfer fritters to plate lined with kitchen paper towels to drain.

6. Serve immediately with lemon wedges.

Nutrition:

Calories: 271

Carbohydrates: 3.5g

Proteins: 16g

Fat: 22g

Fiber: 1g

114. Mussels with Herbed Butter on Grill

Preparation Time: 15 minutes

Cooking Time: 10 minutes

Servings: 4

Ingredients:

- 1/2 cup of butter unsalted, softened
- 2 Tbsp fresh parsley, chopped
- 1 Tbsp of fresh dill
- 2 Tbsp of spring/green onions finely chopped
- 2 tsp lemon juice
- Salt and freshly ground pepper
- 2 lbs. of fresh mussels
- Lemon For serving

Directions:

1. In a bowl, combine butter, softened at room temperature, parsley, dill, spring onions and lemon juice.

2. Season with the salt and pepper to taste.

3. Preheat your grill (pellet, gas, charcoal) to HIGH according to manufacturer Instructions.

4. Grill mussels for 8 - 10 minutes or until shells open.

5. Remove mussels on serving plate, pour with herbed butter, and serve with lemon.

Nutrition:

Calories: 401 Carbohydrates: 8g

Proteins: 28g Fat: 29g

Fiber: 0.3g

115. Mussels with Saffron

Preparation Time: 5 minutes

Cooking Time: 8 minutes

Servings: 4

Ingredients:

- 2 lbs. of mussels, cleaned
- 1 onion, finely chopped
- 4 Tbsp heavy cream
- 1/2 cup of dry white wine
- Pepper to taste
- 1 pinch of saffron
- 2 Tbsp of fresh parsley, finely chopped

Directions:

1. In a large pot, boil the mussels with white wine, chopped onion and ground black pepper.

2. In a separate saucepot, boil the cream with a pinch of saffron for 2 minutes.

3. Drain the mussels and combine with the cream and saffron.

4. Serve immediately with parsley.

Nutrition:

Calories: 259

Carbohydrates: 9g

Proteins: 28g

Fat: 8g

Fiber: 0.6g

116. Hearty Meatballs

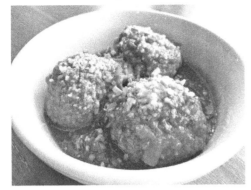

Preparation Time: 10 minutes

Cooking Time: 20 minutes

Servings: 6

Ingredients:

For Meatball:

- 1 tablespoon lemon juice
- ¼ teaspoon dry mustard
- ¾ teaspoon onion powder
- 1 teaspoon Italian seasoning
- 1 teaspoon poultry seasoning, unsalted
- 1 teaspoon black pepper
- 1-pound lean ground beef or turkey
- ¼ cup onion, finely chopped
- 1 teaspoon granulated sugar

1 teaspoon Tabasco sauce

For Sauce:

- 1 teaspoon onion powder
- 2 teaspoons vinegar
- 2 teaspoons sugar
- ¼ cup of vegetable oil
- 2 tablespoons all-purpose flour
- 1 teaspoon Tabasco sauce
- 2-3 cups water

Directions:

1. Preheat an oven to 425 **degree** F. Grease a baking dish with some cooking spray.

2. In a mixing bowl, add all meatball ingredients. Combine to mix well with each other.

3. Prepare meatballs from it and bake in a baking dish for 20 minutes until evenly brown.

4. Take a medium saucepan or skillet, add oil. Heat over medium heat.

5. Add flour, vinegar, sugar, onion powder, mild sauce, and water; stir-cook until sauce thickens.

6. Serve meatballs with sauce on top.

Nutrition:

Calories: 176 Fat: 11g

Phosphorus: 91mg

Potassium: 152mg

Sodium: 61mg

Carbohydrates: 6g

Protein: 14g

117. Broiled Lamb Chops

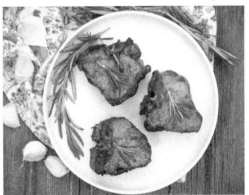

Preparation Time: 10 minutes

Cooking Time: 2 hours and 10 minutes

Servings: 6

Ingredients:

- 4 to 6 lamb loin chops
- 10 to 12 sprigs of fresh rosemary
- Four large garlic cloves halved
- 3 tablespoons of good olive oil

- 2 teaspoons of sea salt (fine)
- 1/2 teaspoon of black pepper (freshly ground)

Directions:

1. Set the oven to broil.

2. Place the seasoned chops on a sheet pan that has been greased. Insert the sliced garlic cloves into the lamb chops.

3. Remove the leaves from the rosemary plant by placing one hand near the top of the stem and then use your fingers on the opposite hand to scrape down the entire stem from the top to the base. Or, you can simply leave the sprig whole to make it easier to remove later.

4. Take the fresh rosemary leaves and gently roll them between your hands' palms to release their natural oils.

5. Next, place a few of the freshly pressed rosemary leaves, or the just the whole spring, on top of each of the chops.

6. Place the lamb chops into the oven to be at least 8 or more inches from the heat source.

7. Allow the lamb chops to broil until they are perfectly medium-rare, or about 8 minutes. For rare chops, about 6 minutes, or about 12 minutes for well-done chops.

8. When you are ready to eat the lamb chops, simply remove the garlic halves, brush the rosemary aside with your utensil, and then dig in.

9. Large chunks of cooked garlic can be a bit overpowering to some people. At the same time, rosemary, whether fresh or dry, tends to have a woodsy texture that can make it tough to chew.

10. Therefore, you'll want to remove them before indulging in your lamb chops for best results.

Nutrition:

Calories: 169.6 kcal

Total Fat: 5.9 g

Saturated Fat: 2.3 g

Cholesterol: 72.6 mg

Sodium: 657.6 mg

Total Carbs: 8.3 g

Fiber: 3.2 g

Sugar: 0.4 g

Protein: 24.1 g

118. Healthy Sweet Potato Puree

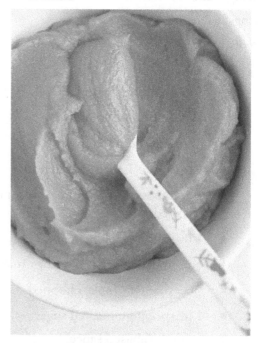

Preparation Time: 10 minutes

Cooking Time: 1 hour

Servings: 8

Ingredients:

- 1/2 cup buttermilk
- 1/2 cup whole milk6 tablespoons butter

Directions:

1. Adjust oven rack to upper-middle position; heat to 425 degrees. Place potatoes on a foil-lined pan; bake 45 to

60 minutes, until tender. Peel when cool enough to handle.

2. Puree with salt and pepper in a food processor. With motor running, gradually add milks through feeder tube, then butter.

3. Process until silken. (Can make up to 2 days ahead; store in an airtight container.) Reheat and serve.

Nutrition:

Calories: 238 kcal

Total Fat: 9.4 g

Saturated Fat: 0 g

Cholesterol: 25 mg

Sodium: 323 mg

Total Carbs: 3.7 g

Fiber: 0 g

Sugar: 0 g

Protein: 3.8 g

119. Hearty Chicken Rice Combo

Preparation Time: 10 minutes

Cooking Time: 10 minutes

Servings: 6

Ingredients:

- 12 ounces boneless, skinless chicken breast, cut into 12 strips
- Cooked white rice
- Juice of 2 limes
- 2 tablespoons brown sugar
- 1 tablespoon minced garlic
- 2 teaspoons ground cumin

Directions:

1. In a mixing bowl, add lime juice, brown sugar, garlic, and cumin. Combine to mix well with each other.

2. Add chicken and combine well. Marinate for 1 hour in the refrigerator.

3. Remove chicken and thread into pre-soaked skewers.

4. Preheat grill over medium heat setting; grease grates with some oil.

5. Grill chicken 4 minutes each side until golden brown and juicy.

6. Serve warm with cooked rice.

Nutrition:

Calories: 93

Fat: 2g

Phosphorus: 131mg

Potassium: 233mg

Sodium: 110mg

Carbohydrates: 5g

Protein: 12g

CHAPTER 7:

Snacks

120. Asian Pear Salad

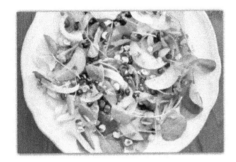

Preparation time: 10 minutes

Cooking time: 5 minutes

Servings: 6

Ingredients:

- ½ cup sugar
- ½ cup water
- ½ cup walnuts or pecans
- 6 cups green leaf lettuce
- 4 Asian pears, peeled, cored, and diced
- 2 ounces stilton or blue cheese
- ½ cup pomegranate seeds
- Vinegar dressing

Directions:

1. Prepare the sugar syrup by cooking sugar with water in a non-stick pan.
2. Cook until it thickens, then stir in nuts.
3. Layer a baking sheet with aluminum foil and pour the nut mixture over it.

4. Transfer the nuts to a bowl and add lettuce, cheese, pears, and pomegranate seeds.
5. Whisk the vinegar dressing ingredients in a small bowl.
6. Pour this dressing into the pears salad and mix well.
7. Serve.

Nutrition:

Calories: 301 Carbohydrates: 41 g Protein: 6 g

Dietary Fiber: 14 g Sodium: 206 mg

Potassium: 297 mg Phosphorus: 127 mg

121. Queso Dip

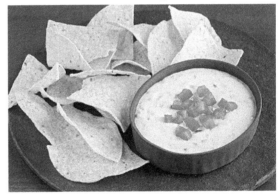

Preparation Time: 10 minutes

Cooking Time: 10 minutes

Servings: 4

Ingredients:

- 1/2 cup roasted tomatoes, diced
- 1/4 teaspoon ground cumin
- 4 oz can green chili peppers, diced
- 1/4 cup heavy cream

96 | P a g .

- 1/2 lb. white American cheese, diced

Directions:

1. Add heavy cream and cheese to the saucepan and heat over medium-low heat until cheese is melted.

2. Remove saucepan from heat. Add remaining ingredients and stir everything well.

3. Serve and enjoy.

Nutrition:

Calories 261 Fat 21.1 g

Carbohydrates 6.9 g

Sugar 4.8 g Protein 10.8 g

Cholesterol 61 mg

122.   Jalapeno Salsa

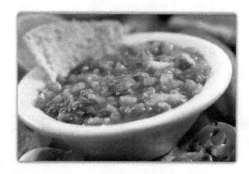

Preparation time: 10 minutes

Cooking time: 0 minutes

Servings: 8

Ingredients:

- 4 Roma tomatoes, chopped
- 2 green onions, chopped
- 3 garlic cloves, minced
- 1 green bell pepper, chopped
- 1 fresh jalapeño, chopped
- ½ bunch fresh cilantro, chopped
- ½ teaspoon cumin
- ¼ cup fresh oregano, chopped

Directions:

1. Add bell pepper, jalapeno, cilantro, tomatoes, onion, and all other ingredients to a blender.

2. Blend this salsa mixture until it gets chunky.

3. Serve fresh.

Nutrition:

Calories: 14 Carbohydrates: 2 g

Protein: 1 g Dietary Fiber: 0 g Fat: 1 g

Sodium: 4 mg Potassium: 117 mg

Phosphorus: 14 mg

123.   Kale Spread

Preparation Time: 10 minutes

Cooking Time: 5 minutes

Servings: 10

Ingredients:

- 6 cups kale, chopped
- 1/2 cup hemp hearts
- 1/2 cup olive oil
- 1 tablespoon olive oil
- 1/2 cup green onions
- 3 tablespoon apple cider vinegar
- 1 1/4 teaspoon sea salt

Directions:

1. Heat oil in a pan over low heat.

2. Add kale and sauté for 5-7 minutes.

3. Transfer kale into a food processor along with remaining ingredients and process until smooth.

4. Serve and enjoy.

Nutrition:

Calories 166 Fat 15 g

Carbohydrates 6 g Sugar 0.3 g

Protein 4 g Cholesterol 0 mg

124. Lemon Cauliflower Hummus

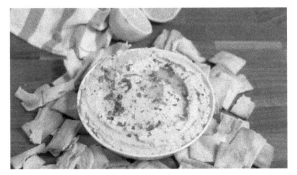

Preparation Time: 10 minutes

Cooking Time: 5 minutes

Servings: 6

Ingredients:

- 3 cups cauliflower florets
- 1 1/2 tablespoon tahini paste
- 2 tablespoon olive oil
- 2 garlic cloves
- 3 tablespoon fresh lemon juice
- 1/2 teaspoon salt

Directions:

1. Add cauliflower into the boiling water and cook for 10-15 minutes or until softened. Drain well.

2. Transfer cauliflower into the blender along with remaining ingredients and blend until smooth.

3. Serve and enjoy.

Nutrition:

Calories 105

Fat 9 g

Carbohydrates 4 g

Sugar 1 g

Protein 2 g

Cholesterol 0 mg

125. Sweet Peanut Butter Dip

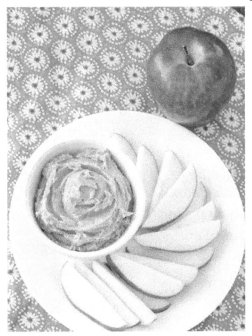

Preparation Time: 5 minutes

Cooking Time: 5 minutes

Servings: 6

Ingredients:

- 1/2 cup peanut butter
- 1/3 cup unsweetened almond milk
- 1 teaspoon vanilla
- 30 drops liquid stevia

Directions:

1. Add all ingredients in a bowl and mix until well combined.

2. Serve and enjoy.

Nutrition:

Calories 131

Fat 11 g

Carbohydrates 4 g

Sugar 2 g

Protein 6 g

Cholesterol 0 mg

126. Chili Cheese Dip

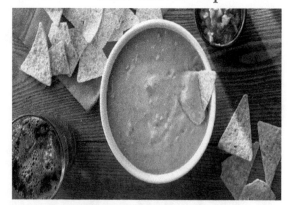

Preparation Time: 10 minutes

Cooking Time: 6 hours

Servings: 8

Ingredients:

- 4 oz can green chilies, diced
- 2 cups fresh tomatoes, diced
- 1 onion, chopped
- 1 3/4 cups cheese, cubed

Directions:

1. Add all ingredients into the crockpot and stir well.
2. Cover and cook on low for 6 hours.
3. Stir and serve.

Nutrition:

Calories 105

Fat 7 g

Carbohydrates 4 g

Sugar 2 g

Protein 6 g

Cholesterol 20 mg

127. Delicious Tzatziki

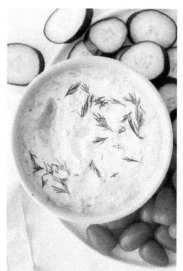

Preparation Time: 5 minutes

Cooking Time: 5 minutes

Servings: 4

Ingredients:

- 1 cup cucumber, grated and squeeze out all liquid
- 2 tablespoon fresh dill, chopped
- 1/2 cup sour cream
- 1/2 cup yogurt
- 1 tablespoon fresh lemon juice
- 1 garlic clove, minced
- 2 teaspoon olive oil
- Pepper
- Salt

Directions:

1. Add all ingredients into the bowl and mix until well to combine.
2. Place in a refrigerator for 2 hours.
3. Serve and enjoy.

Nutrition:

Calories 100 Fat 9 g Carbohydrates 5 g

Sugar 2 g Protein 1 g

Cholesterol 0 mg

128.   Spicy Mexican Salsa

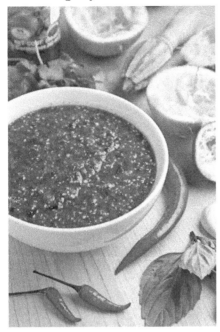

Preparation Time: 5 minutes

Cooking Time: 5 minutes

Servings: 4

Ingredients:

- 4 tomatoes, diced
- 1 jalapeno pepper, diced
- 1/4 onion, chopped
- 2 tablespoon fresh cilantro, chopped
- Pepper
- Salt

Directions:

1. Add all ingredients into the bowl and mix well.
2. Serve and enjoy.

Nutrition:

Calories 25

Fat 0.5 g

Carbohydrates 6 g

Sugar 3 g

Protein 1 g

Cholesterol 0 mg

129.   Pecan Caramel Corn

Preparation time: 10 minutes

Cooking time: 1 hour, 5 minutes

Servings: 10

Ingredients:

- 20 cups popped popcorn
- 2 cups unblanched almonds
- 1 cup pecan halves
- 1 cup granulated sugar
- 1 cup unsalted butter
- ½ cup corn syrup
- Pinch of cream of tartar
- 1 teaspoon baking soda

Directions:

1. Take a large roasting pan and layer it with popcorn, almonds, and pecans.
2. Cook sugar with corn syrup, butter, and cream of tartar in a heavy saucepan.
3. Stir this syrup for 5 minutes on a boil, then stir in baking soda.
4. Pour this caramel sauce over the popcorn and almonds in the pan.
5. Bake the almonds and popcorn for 1 hour at 200°F in the oven.
6. Stir well, then serve.

Nutrition:

Calories: 604

Carbohydrates: 51 g

Protein: 8 g

Dietary Fiber: 4 g

Fat: 6 g

Sodium: 149 mg

Potassium: 285 mg

Phosphorus: 201 mg

130. Flavors BLT Dip

Preparation Time: 10 minutes

Cooking Time: 10 minutes

Servings: 12

Ingredients:

- 1 lb. bacon, cooked and chopped
- 1 cup tomato, chopped
- 1 cup lettuce, chopped
- 1/2 teaspoon paprika
- 1 teaspoon garlic, minced
- 1 teaspoon onion powder
- 1/4 cup cheddar cheese, shredded
- 1/4 cup sour cream
- 1/4 cup mayonnaise
- 8 oz cream cheese

Directions:

1. Add all ingredients into the mixing bowl and mix until well combined.
2. Serve and enjoy.

Nutrition:

Calories 314

Fat 25.9 g

Carbohydrates 3.5 g

Sugar 0.9 g

Protein 16.4 g

Cholesterol 68 mg

131. Cocoa Vanilla Nuts

Preparation time: 2 minutes

Cooking time: 1 hour

Servings: 6

Ingredients:

- ½ cup pecan halves
- ½ cup walnuts halves
- ½ cup slivered almonds
- 2 tablespoon cocoa powder, unsweetened
- 1 tablespoon vanilla extract
- 2 tablespoon swerve
- 2 tablespoon butter, unsalted and melted

Directions:

1. Add all the ingredients in your slow cooker and stir well to combine.
2. Cover the slow cooker and cook on high for 1 hour.
3. When the time has elapsed, transfer the nuts to a baking sheet to cool.
4. Serve and enjoy or store in airtight containers.

Nutrition:

Calories 225,

Total Fat 21g,

Saturated Fat 4g,

Total Carbs 5g,

Net Carbs 2g,

Protein 4g,

Sugar: 1g,

Fiber: 2g,

Sodium: 1mg,

Potassium 171g

132. Cucumber Cream Cheese Frosting Cake

Preparation time: 45 minutes

Cooking time: 3 hours

Servings: 12

Ingredients:

- ¼ cup coconut oil
- 1 ½ cup almond flour
- ¾ cup swerve
- ½ cup coconut, shredded

- ½ cup walnuts or pecans, chopped
- 2 tablespoon baking powder
- ¼ cup whey protein powder, unflavored
- 1 tablespoon cinnamon, ground
- ¼ tablespoon garlic cloves, ground
- ¼ tablespoon salt
- 2 cups cucumbers, grated
- 4 eggs
- 3 tablespoon almond milk
- ½ tablespoon vanilla extract
- Cream Cheese Frosting
- ½ cup swerve
- 6 oz cream cheese, softened
- ¾ tablespoon vanilla extract
- ½ cup heavy cream

Directions:

1. Grease your 6-quart slow cooker inside and line with parchment paper ensuring you put plenty of parchment paper on the sides. Grease the parchment paper with coconut oil too.

2. Whisk together flour, swerve sweetener, coconut, walnuts, baking powder, protein powder, cinnamon, garlic and salt in a large mixing bowl.

3. Stir in cucumber, eggs, coconut oil, milk, and vanilla extract. Mix until well combined then spread the batter in the slow cooker.

4. Cook on low for 3 hours. Once time has elapsed, let the cake rest to cool completely then lift it out of the slow cooker and place it on a platter.

5. Meanwhile, prepare the frosting by beating sweetener with cream cheese until smooth.

6. Beat in vanilla extract until smooth then spread the mixture over the cake.

7. Slice the cake, serve and enjoy.

Nutrition:

Calories 351.18, Total Fat 30.62g,

Saturated Fat 16.3g,

Total Carbs 9.5g,

Protein 9.4g,

Sugar: 11g,

Fiber: 4.14g,

Sodium: 229mg

133. Corned Beef Mixed Cheese

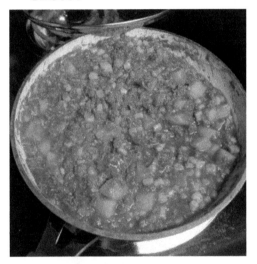

Preparation time: 5 minutes

Cooking Time: 3 hours

Servings: 5

Ingredients:

- 2½ cups corned beef, cubed and cooked
- 1, 14-ounces, can rinsed and drained sauerkraut
- 2 cups Swiss cheese, shredded
- 2 cups cheddar cheese, shredded
- 1 cup mayonnaise

Directions:

1. Combine beef, sauerkraut, Swiss cheese, cheddar cheese and mayonnaise in a slow cooker then cover.
2. Cook for about 3-4 hours until cheese melts and it's heated through.
3. Serve and enjoy

Nutrition:

Calories: 101,

Total fat: 9g,

Saturated fat: 3g,

Total carbs: 1g,

Protein: 4g,

Sugars: 0g,

Fiber: 0g,

Sodium: 233mg,

Potassium: 197mg

134. Chicken Cheese Dip

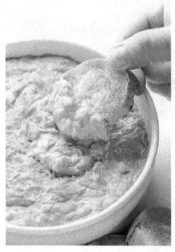

Preparation Time: 10 minutes

Cooking Time: 2 hours

Servings: 10

Ingredients:

- 1/2 lb. cheese, cubed
- 1 cup cooked chicken, shredded

- 1/2 cup bell peppers, chopped
- 10 oz can tomato with green chilies

Directions:

1. Add all ingredients into the crockpot and stir well.
2. Cover and cook on low for 2 hours.
3. Stir and serve.

Nutrition:

Calories 121 Fat 7 g

Carbohydrates 3 g Sugar 0.5 g

Protein 11 g Cholesterol 36 mg

135. Kale Chips

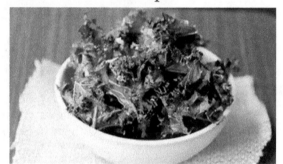

Preparation time: 20 minutes

Cooking time: 25 minutes

Servings: 6

Ingredients:

- Kale – 2 cups
- Olive oil – 2 teaspoon.
- Chili powder – ¼ teaspoon.
- Pinch cayenne pepper

Directions:

1. Preheat the oven to 300F.
2. Line 2 baking sheets with parchment paper; set aside.
3. Remove the stems from the kale and tear the leaves into 2-inch pieces.
4. Wash the kale and dry it completely.

5. Transfer the kale to a large bowl and drizzle with olive oil.

6. Use your hands to toss the kale with oil, taking care to coat each leaf evenly.

7. Season the kale with chili powder and cayenne pepper and toss to combine thoroughly.

8. Spread the seasoned kale in a single layer on each baking sheet. Do not overlap the leaves.

9. Bake the kale, rotating the pans once, for 20 to 25 minutes until it is crisp and dry.

10. Remove the trays from the oven and allow the chips to cool on the trays for 5 minutes.

Nutrition:

Calories: 24 Fat: 2g Carb: 2g

Phosphorus: 21mg Potassium: 111mg

Sodium: 13mg Protein: 1g

Directions:

1. Preheat the oven to 350F.

2. Line a baking sheet with parchment paper.

3. In a small bowl, stir together the sugar, cinnamon, and nutmeg.

4. Lay the tortillas on a clean work surface and spray both sides of each lightly with cooking spray.

5. Sprinkle the cinnamon sugar evenly over both sides of each tortilla.

6. Cut the tortillas into 16 wedges each and place them on the baking sheet.

7. Bake the tortilla wedges, turning once, for about 10 minutes or until crisp.

8. Cool the chips serve.

Nutrition:

Calories: 51 Fat: 1g Carb: 9g

Phosphorus: 29mg Potassium: 24mg

Sodium: 103 mg Protein: 1g

136.   Tortilla Chips

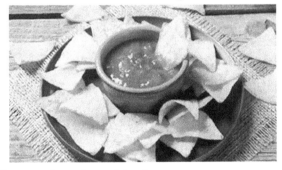

Preparation time: 15 minutes

Cooking time: 10 minutes

Servings: 6

Ingredients:

- Granulated sugar – 2 teaspoons.

- Ground cinnamon – ½ teaspoon.

- Pinch ground nutmeg

- Flour tortillas – 3 (6-inch)

- Cooking spray

137.   Corn Bread

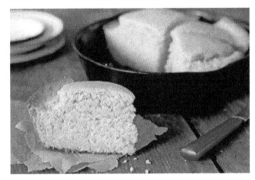

Preparation time: 10 minutes

Cooking time: 20 minutes

Servings: 10

Ingredients:

- Cooking spray for greasing the baking dish

- Yellow cornmeal – 1 ¼ cups

- All-purpose flour – ¾ cup

- Baking soda substitute – 1 tablespoon.
- Granulated sugar – ½ cup
- Eggs – 2
- Unsweetened, unfortified rice milk – 1 cup
- Olive oil – 2 Tablespoons.

Directions:

1. Preheat the oven to 425F.
2. Lightly spray an 8-by-8-inch baking dish with cooking spray. Set aside.
3. In a medium bowl, stir together the cornmeal, flour, baking soda substitute, and sugar.
4. In a small bowl, whisk together the eggs, rice milk, and olive oil until blended.
5. Add the wet ingredients to the dry ingredients and stir until well combined.
6. Pour the batter into the baking dish and bake for 20 minutes or until golden and cooked through.
7. Serve warm.

Nutrition:

Calories: 198 Fat: 5g Carb: 34g

Phosphorus: 88mg Potassium: 94mg

Sodium: 25mg Protein: 4g

138. Vegetable Rolls

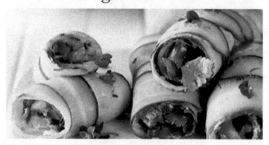

Preparation time: 30 minutes

Cooking time: 0 minutes

Servings: 8

Ingredients:

- Finely shredded red cabbage – ½ cup
- Grated carrot – ½ cup
- Julienne red bell pepper – ¼ cup
- Julienned scallion – ¼ cup, both green and white parts
- Chopped cilantro – ¼ cup
- Olive oil – 1 Tablespoon.
- Ground cumin – ¼ teaspoon.
- Freshly ground black pepper – ¼ teaspoon.
- English cucumber – 1, sliced very thin strips

Directions:

1. In a bowl, toss together the black pepper, cumin, olive oil, cilantro, scallion, red pepper, carrot, and cabbage. Mix well.
2. Evenly divide the vegetable filling among the cucumber strips, placing the filling close to one end of the strip.
3. Roll up the cucumber strips around the filling and secure with a wooden pick.
4. Repeat with each cucumber strip.

Nutrition:

Calories: 26

Fat: 2g

Carb: 3g

Phosphorus: 14mg

Potassium: 95mg

Sodium: 7mg

Protein: 0g

139. Frittata with Penne

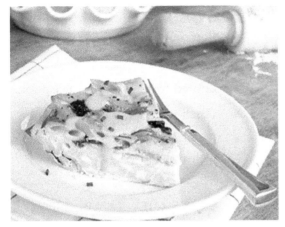

Preparation time: 15 minutes

Cooking time: 30 minutes

Servings: 4

Ingredients:

- Egg whites- 6
- Rice milk – ¼ cup
- Chopped fresh parsley – 1 Tablespoon.
- Chopped fresh thyme – 1 teaspoon.
- Chopped fresh chives – 1 teaspoon.
- Ground black pepper
- Olive oil – 2 teaspoons.
- Small sweet onion – ¼, chopped
- Minced garlic – 1 teaspoon.
- Boiled and chopped red bell pepper – ½ cup
- Cooked penne – 2 cups

Directions:

1. Preheat the oven to 350F.
2. In a bowl, whisk together the egg whites, rice milk, parsley, thyme, chives, and pepper.
3. Heat the oil in a skillet.
4. Sauté the onion, garlic, red pepper for 4 minutes or until they are softened.

5. Add the cooked penne to the skillet.
6. Pour the egg mixture over the pasta and shake the pan to coat the pasta.
7. Leave the skillet on the heat for 1 minute to set the bottom of the frittata and then transfer the skillet to the oven.
8. Bake, the frittata for 25 minutes or until it is set and golden brown.
9. Serve.

Nutrition:

Calories: 170 Fat: 3g Carb: 25g

Phosphorus: 62mg Potassium: 144mg

Sodium: 90mg Protein: 10g

140. Vegetable Fried Rice

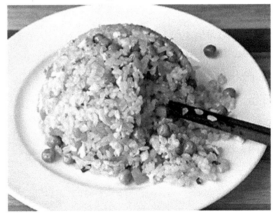

Preparation time: 20 minutes

Cooking time: 20 minutes

Servings: 6

Ingredients:

- Olive oil – 1 Tablespoon.
- Sweet onion – ½, chopped
- Grated fresh ginger – 1 Tablespoon.
- Minced garlic - 2 teaspoons.
- Sliced carrots – 1 cup
- Chopped eggplant – ½ cup
- Peas – ½ cup

- Green beans – ½ cup, cut into 1-inch pieces
- Chopped fresh cilantro – 2 Tablespoon.
- Cooked rice – 3 cups

Directions:

1. Heat the olive oil in a skillet.
2. Sauté the ginger, onion, and garlic for 3 minutes or until softened.
3. Stir in carrot, eggplant, green beans, and peas and sauté for 3 minutes more.
4. Add cilantro and rice.
5. Sauté, continually stirring, for about 10 minutes or until the rice is heated through.
6. Serve.

Nutrition:

Calories: 189 Fat: 7g Carb: 28g

Phosphorus: 89mg Potassium: 172mg

Sodium: 13mg Protein: 6g

141.   Tofu Stir-Fry

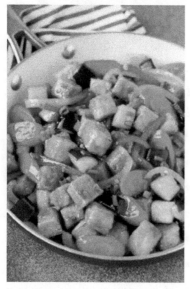

Preparation time: 20 minutes

Cooking time: 20 minutes

Servings: 4

Ingredients:

For the tofu

- Lemon juice – 1 Tablespoon.
- Minced garlic – 1 teaspoon.
- Grated fresh ginger – 1 teaspoon.
- Pinch red pepper flakes
- Extra-firm tofu- 5 ounces, pressed well and cubed

For the stir-fry

- OLIVE OIL – 1 TABLESPOON.
- CAULIFLOWER FLORETS – ½ CUP
- THINLY SLICED CARROTS – ½ CUP
- JULIENNED RED PEPPER – ½ CUP
- FRESH GREEN BEANS – ½ CUP
- Cooked white rice – 2 cups

Directions:

1. In a bowl, mix the lemon juice, garlic, ginger, and red pepper flakes.
2. Add the tofu and toss to coat.
3. Place the bowl in the refrigerator and marinate for 2 hours.
4. To make the stir-fry, heat the oil in a skillet. Sauté the tofu for 8 minutes or until it is lightly browned and heated through.
5. Add the carrots, and cauliflower and sauté for 5 minutes. Stirring and tossing constantly.
6. Add the red pepper and green beans, sauté for 3 minutes more.
7. Serve over white rice.

Nutrition:

Calories: 190 Fat: 6g Carb: 30g

Phosphorus: 90mg Potassium: 199mg

Sodium: 22mg Protein: 6g

142. Lasagna

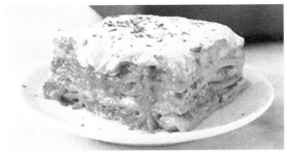

Preparation time: 10 minutes

Cooking time: 1 hour

Servings: 2

Ingredients:

- Soft tofu - ½ pack
- Baby spinach – ½ cup
- Unenriched rick milk – 4 Tablespoons.
- Garlic – 1 clove, crushed
- Lemon – 1, juiced
- Fresh basil – 2 Tablespoons. chopped
- A pinch of black pepper to taste
- Zucchini – 1, sliced
- Red bell pepper – 1, sliced
- Eggplant – 1 sliced

Directions:

1. Preheat the oven to 325F. Soak vegetables in warm water before cooking.
2. In a blender, process the tofu, garlic, milk, basil, lemon juice, and pepper until smooth.
3. Toss in the zucchini and spinach for the last 30 seconds.
4. Layer the bottom of the dish with 1/3 eggplant slices and 1/3 red pepper slices and then cover with 1/3 of the tofu sauce. Repeat to complete.

5. Bake in the oven for 1 hour or until the vegetables are soft through to the center.
6. Finish under the broiler until golden and bubbly.
7. Divide into portions and serve with a sprinkle of black pepper to taste.

Nutrition:

Calories: 116

Fat: 4g

Carb: 10g

Phosphorus: 149mg

Potassium: 346mg

Sodium: 27mg

Protein: 5g

143. Cauliflower Patties

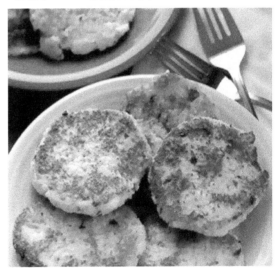

Preparation time: 5 minutes

Cooking time: 8 minutes

Servings: 2

Ingredients:

- Eggs – 2
- Egg whites – 2
- Onion – ½, diced
- Cauliflower – 2 cups, frozen

- All-purpose white flour – 2 Tablespoons.

- Black pepper – 1 teaspoon.

- Coconut oil – 1 Tablespoon.

- Curry powder – 1 teaspoon.

- Fresh cilantro – 1 Tablespoon.

Directions:

1. Soak vegetables in warm water prior to cooking.

2. Steam cauliflower over a pan of boiling water for 10 minutes.

3. Blend eggs and onion in a food processor before adding cooked cauliflower, spices, cilantro, flour, and pepper and blast in the processor for 30 seconds.

4. Heat a skillet on a high heat and add oil.

5. Pour tablespoon. portions of the cauliflower mixture into the pan and brown on each side until crispy, about 3 to 4 minutes.

6. Enjoy with a salad.

Nutrition:

Calories: 227 Fat: 12g Carb: 15g

Phosphorus: 193mg Potassium: 513mg

Sodium: 158mg Protein: 13g

144.   Turnip Chips

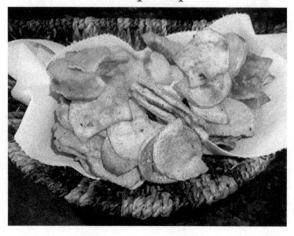

Preparation time: 5 minutes

Cooking time: 50 minutes

Servings: 2

Ingredients:

- Turnips – 2, peeled and sliced

- Extra virgin olive oil – 1 Tablespoon.

- Onion – 1 chopped

- Minced garlic – 1 clove

- Black pepper – 1 teaspoon.

- Oregano – 1 teaspoon.

- Paprika - 1 teaspoon.

Directions:

1. Preheat oven to 375F. Grease a baking tray with olive oil.

2. Add turnip slices in a thin layer.

3. Dust over herbs and spices with an extra drizzle of olive oil.

4. Bake 40 minutes. Turning once.

Nutrition:

Calories: 136 Fat: 14g

Carb: 30g

Phosphorus: 50mg

Potassium: 356mg

Sodium: 71mg

Protein: g

145.   Flovers Nacho Dip

Preparation Time: 10 minutes

Cooking Time: 2 hours

Servings: 8

Ingredients:

- 8 oz cream cheese

- 1/2 cup salsa

- 1 cup cheddar cheese, shredded

- 1/4 cup unsweetened almond milk

Directions:

1. Add all ingredients into the crockpot and stir well.
2. Cover and cook on low for 2 hours.
3. Stir well and serve.

Nutrition:

Calories 175

Fat 16 g

Carbohydrates 2 g

Sugar 1 g

Protein 6 g

Cholesterol 45 mg

146.   Beef Dip

Preparation Time: 10 minutes

Cooking Time: 60 minutes

Servings: 20

Ingredients:

- 2 lbs. ground beef
- 2 kg. cheese, cubed
- 30 oz salsa

Directions:

1. Heat pan over medium heat.
2. Add meat and cook until beef is browned.
3. Transfer browned meat into the crockpot.
4. Add remaining ingredients and stir well.
5. Cover and cook on high for 1 hour.
6. Stir well and serve.

Nutrition:

Calories 280 Fat 18 g

Carbohydrates 3 g

Sugar 1 g

Protein 25 g

Cholesterol 85 mg

147.   Sweet Apricot Glazed Party Meatballs

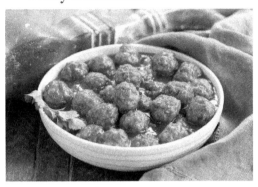

Preparation time: 20 minutes

Cooking time: 3 hours

Servings: 9

Ingredients:

For Meatballs

- 1 ½ lb. beef, ground
- ½ lb. pork, ground
- 3 tablespoon onions, finely diced
- 2 eggs
- ¼ cup heavy cream
- 2 tablespoon dried parsley
- 2 tablespoon salt
- ½ tablespoon black pepper
- ¼ tablespoon nutmeg

For the Glaze:

- ½ cup Smuckers Apricot preserves, sugar-free
- ½ cup BBQ sauce, sugar-free
- 1 tablespoon soy sauce
- 3 tablespoon chili garlic sauce

Directions:

1. Preheat oven to 4000F. Line a baking sheet with foil and set aside.
2. For the glaze
3. Blend all the glaze ingredients until well combined then set aside.
4. For the meatballs

5. Add all the ingredients in a mixing bowl and use a hand mixer or your hands to mix until well combined.

6. Take a tablespoon size of the mixture and mold it into meatballs.

7. Place the meatballs on the prepared baking sheet.

8. Place the baking sheet at the center rack of your preheated oven and bake for 15 minutes.

9. Transfer the meatballs to your slow cooker and pour the glaze on top.

10. Carefully mix the meatballs into the glaze, cover and cook on low for six hours stirring occasionally.

11. Let the meatballs sit to cool before serving.

Nutrition:

Calories 308, Total Fat 20g, Saturated Fat 7g,

Total Carbs 6g, Net Carbs 4g, Protein 26g,

Sugar: 2g, Fiber: 2g

148. Date and Blueberry Muffins

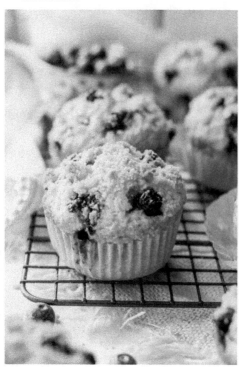

Preparation time: 20 minutes

Cooking time: 30 minutes

Servings: 12

Ingredients:

- 2 tablespoons flax meal
- 6 tablespoons water
- 1 cup almond flour
- 1 cup coconut flour
- 2 teaspoons baking soda
- 1 teaspoon sea salt
- 2 tablespoons mixed spice
- 1 cup dates, pitted
- 2 cups canned pumpkin
- 1 teaspoon lemon juice
- ¼ cup coconut oil
- 5 ounces frozen blueberries
- ¾ cup zucchini, grated
- ¾ cup chopped walnuts

Directions:

1. Preheat oven to 350° f.

2. Line 12 muffin cups with paper liners.

3. Mix the flax meal and water and leave for a few minutes until it becomes a gel-like consistency.

4. Mix almond flour, coconut flour, baking soda, sea salt and mixed spice in large bowl. Set aside.

5. In a food processor, pulse together the pitted dates, pumpkin and lemon juice together with the flax water and coconut oil.

6. Add the pumpkin mix into the dry ingredients. Mix well.

7. Gently stir in the blueberries, grated zucchini and walnuts.

8. Divide the mixture evenly between the prepared muffin cups.

9. Bake for about 30 minutes. If the muffins are too gooey, after this time, leave for a few minutes longer.

Nutrition:

Calories 211,

Fat 12.0g,

Carbs 23.3g,

Dietary fiber 7.2g,

Protein 5.0g

149. Cranberry and Lemon Cookies

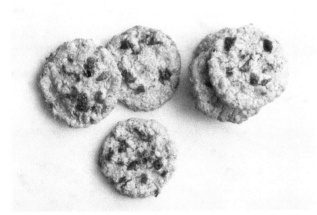

Preparation time: 20 minutes

Cooking time: 15 minutes

Servings: 12

Ingredients:

- ½ cup coconut milk
- 1 tablespoon ground flaxseed
- 1¼ cups brown organic superfine sugar
- ½ cup unsweetened apple sauce
- ¼ cup vegetable oil
- 1 tablespoon fresh lemon juice
- 1½ teaspoons lemon zest
- 2 teaspoons vanilla extract
- 1¼ cups unbleached general-purpose flour
- 1 cup whole wheat flour

- 1 teaspoon baking soda ½ teaspoon salt
- 1 cup dried cranberries
- 1 cup chopped walnuts

Directions:

1. Pre-heat the oven to 350°f.
2. Prepare 2 cookie sheets with parchment paper.
3. Warm the coconut milk and stir in the flaxseed. Leave to one side for it to gel.
4. In a large bowl, stir together all of the wet ingredients with the sugar. Stir in the gelled flax seed.
5. In another bowl sift together the flours, baking soda and salt.
6. Put the flour mix to the wet ingredients a little at a time until fully combined.
7. When a dough has formed stir in the nuts and cranberries.
8. Using a spoon form 2-inch round cookies on the prepared sheets.
9. Bake for 12 – 15 minutes until a nice golden brown.
10. Take away from the oven and let it rest on the cookie sheet for about 5 minutes. Place on a cooling rack.
11. Serve, eat and enjoy!

Nutrition:

Calories 332, Fat 13.6g, Carbs 48.8g,

Dietary fiber 2.4g,

Protein 4.9g

150. No Bake Oat Cookies

Preparation time: 30 minutes

Cooking time: 0 minutes

Servings: 24

Ingredients:

- ½ cup plain soymilk
- 1¾ cups sugar

- ½ cup vegan butter
- 1 teaspoon vanilla extract
- 3½ cups quick cooking oats
- ¼ cup unsweetened cocoa powder
- ½ cup smooth or crunchy peanut butter

Directions:

1. In a small pot mix the milk, butter, sugar, peanut butter and vanilla and cook until smooth and creamy
2. In a large bowl combine the oats and cocoa powder.
3. Pour the warm milk mixture over the oats and stir until all the ingredients have combined.
4. Place dollops of mixture onto a waxed paper lined cookie sheet and let cool for about half an hour.

Nutrition:

Calories 171, Fat 6.7g, Carbs 25.5g,

Dietary fiber 2.0g, Protein 3.3g

151. Chocolate Coconut Quinoa Slices

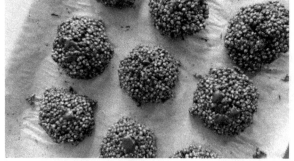

Preparation time: 10 minutes

Cooking time: 25 minutes

Servings: 12

Ingredients:

- ¾ cup quinoa
- ½ cup dried chopped dates
- 3 tablespoons maple syrup

- 2 tablespoons olive oil
- 2 tablespoons ground flaxseed
- ½ teaspoon almond extract
- ¼ teaspoon salt
- ½ cup chocolate protein powder
- ½ cup whole wheat flour
- ¼ cup vegan chocolate chips
- ¼ cup shredded coconut water

Directions:

1. Pre-heat the oven to 350°f.
2. Prepare an 8 x 8 ovenproof baking dish. Grease lightly with oil.
3. Rinse the quinoa in cold water and leave to soak for about 10 minutes.
4. Drain the quinoa. Place 1 cup of water in a small saucepan bring to the boil. Add the quinoa and simmer over a low heat for about 12 minutes. Cool.
5. Mix the cooked quinoa, dates, maple syrup, olive oil, flaxseed, almond extract and salt in a food processor.
6. Process until fairly smooth.
7. In a separate bowl stir together the chocolate protein powder, flour chocolate chips and coconut.
8. Fold the dry mixture into the wet mixture with a flat spatula or knife.
9. Press into the prepared baking dish. Even out the top.
10. Bake for about 25 minutes, until firm.
11. Cool and then slice into bars.
12. Stock in a sealed basin for about a week or freeze up to 3 months.

Nutrition:

Calories 160, Fat 4.7g,

Carbs 22.4g, Dietary fiber 2.9g,

Protein 9.0g

152. Pineapple Raspberry Parfaits

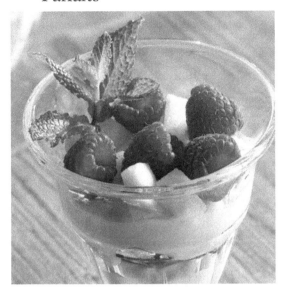

Preparation time: 6 minutes.

Cooking time: 0 minutes.

Servings: 2

Ingredients:

- ½ pint fresh raspberries
- 1 ½ cup fresh or frozen pineapple chunks
- 2 8oz containers non-fat peach yogurt

Directions:

1. In a parfait glass, layer the yogurt, raspberries and pineapples alternately. Chill inside the refrigerator.
2. Serve chilled.

Nutrition:

Calories: 319;

Carbs: 60g;

Protein: 22g;

Fat: 1g;

Phosphorus: 93mg;

Potassium: 479mg;

Sodium: 85mg

153. Cinnamon Apple Chips

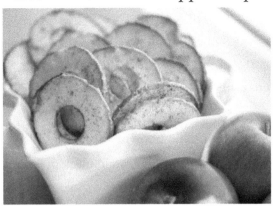

Preparation time: 5 minutes.

Cooking time: 3 hrs.

Servings: 4

Ingredients:

- 4 apples
- 1 teaspoon ground cinnamon

Directions:

1. Preheat the oven to 200°f. Line a baking sheet with parchment paper.
2. Slice the apples into 1/8-inch slices. Toss your cinnamon and apple slices to coat.
3. In a single layer, spread the apples on the prepared baking sheet.
4. Cook for 2 to 3 hours, until the apples are dry. They will still be soft while hot but will crisp once completely cooled.
5. Save in a sealed container for to four days.

Nutrition:

Calories: 96;

Fat: 0g;

Carbs: 26g;

Protein: 1g;

Phosphorus: 0mg;

Potassium: 198mg;

Sodium: 2mg

154. Yogurt Eggplants

Preparation Time: 10 minutes

Cooking Time: 18 minutes

Servings: 4

Ingredients:

- 1 cup Plain yogurt
- 1 tablespoon butter
- 1 teaspoon ground black pepper
- 1 teaspoon salt
- 2 eggplants, chopped
- 1 tablespoon fresh dill, chopped

Directions:

1. Heat butter in the skillet.
2. Toss eggplants in the hot butter. Sprinkle them with salt and ground black pepper.
3. Roast the vegetables for 5 minutes over the medium-high heat. Stir them from time to time.
4. After this, add fresh dill and Plain Yogurt. Mix up well.
5. Close the lid and simmer eggplants for 10 minutes more over the medium-high heat.

Nutrition:

Calories 141, Fat 4.2, Fiber 9.9,

Carbs 21.2, Protein 6.4

155. Roasted Mint Carrots

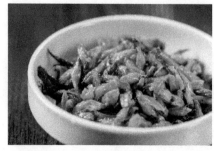

Preparation time: 5 minutes.

Cooking time: 20 minutes.

Servings: 6

Ingredients:

- 1-pound carrots, trimmed
- 1 tablespoon extra-virgin olive oil
- Freshly ground black pepper
- ¼ cup thinly sliced mint

Directions:

1. Preheat the oven to 425°f.
2. In a single layer, arrange the carrots on a rimmed baking sheet. Sprinkle with the olive oil and shake the carrots on the sheet to coat.
3. Season with pepper. Roast for 20 minutes, or until tender and browned, stirring twice while cooking. Sprinkle with the mint and serve.

Nutrition:

Calories: 51; Fat: 2g;

Carbs: 7g; Protein: 1g; Phosphorus: 26mg;

Potassium: 242mg; Sodium: 52mg

156. Walnut Butter on Cracker

Preparation time: 2 minutes.

Cooking time: 0 minutes.

Servings: 1

Ingredients:

- 1 tablespoon walnut butter
- 2 pieces Mary's gone crackers

Directions:

1. Spread ½ tablespoon of walnut butter per cracker and enjoy.

Nutrition:

Calories: 134; Carbs: 4g; Protein: 1g;

Fat: 14g; Phosphorus: 19mg; Potassium: 11mg;

Sodium: 138mg

157. Savory Collard Chips

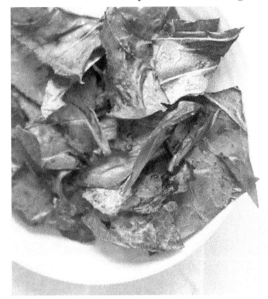

Preparation time: 5 minutes.

Cooking time: 20 minutes.

Servings: 4

Ingredients:

- 1 bunch collard greens
- 1 teaspoon extra-virgin olive oil
- Juice of ½ lemon
- ½ teaspoon garlic powder
- ¼ teaspoon freshly ground black pepper

Directions:

1. Preheat the oven to 350°f. Line a baking sheet with parchment paper.
2. Cut the collards into 2-by-2-inch squares and pat dry with paper towels. In an enormous container, mix the greens with the olive oil, lemon juice, garlic powder, and pepper.
3. Use your hands to mix well, massaging the dressing into the greens until evenly coated.
4. Arrange the collards in a single layer on the baking sheet and cook for 8 minutes. Turn over the pieces and cook for an additional 8 minutes, until crisp.

5. Remove from the oven, let cool, and store in an airtight container in a cool location for up to three days.

Nutrition:

Calories: 24;

Fat: 1g;

Carbs: 3g;

Protein: 1g;

Phosphorus: 6mg;

Potassium: 72mg;

Sodium: 8mg

158. Choco-Chip Cookies with Walnuts and Oatmeal

Preparation time: 20 minutes.

Cooking time: 32 minutes.

Servings: 48

Ingredients:

- ½ cup all-purpose flour
- ½ cup chopped walnuts
- ½ cup whole wheat pastry flour
- ½ teaspoon baking soda
- 1 cup semisweet Choco chip
- 1 large egg
- 1 large egg white
- 1 tablespoon vanilla extract
- 1 teaspoon ground cinnamon
- 2 cups rolled oats (not quick cooking)
- 2/3 cup granulated sugar
- 2/3 cup packed light brown sugar
- 4 tablespoons. Cold unsalted butter, cut into pieces

Directions:

1. Place two racks in the central of the oven, leaving at least a 3-inch space in between them.

2. Preheat oven to 350of and grease baking sheets with cooking spray.

3. In medium bowl, whisk together baking soda, cinnamon, whole wheat flour, all-purpose flour and oats.

4. In a large bowl, with a mixer beat butter until well combined. Add brown sugar and granulated sugar, mixing continuously until creamy.

5. Mix in vanilla, egg white and egg and beat for a minute. Cup by cup mix in the dry ingredients until well incorporated.

6. Fold in walnuts and Choco chips. Get a tablespoon full of the batter and roll with your moistened hands into a ball.

7. Evenly place balls into prepped baking sheets at least 2-inches apart. Place in the oven and bake for 16 minutes.

8. Ten minutes into baking time, switch pans from top to bottom and bottom to top. Continue baking for 6 more minutes.

9. Remove from oven, cool on a wire rack. Allow pans to cool completely before adding the next batch of cookies to be baked.

10. Cookies can be stored for up to 2-weeks in a tightly sealed container or longer in the ref.

Nutrition:

Calories: 71; Carbs: 12g; Protein: 2g;

Fat: 3g; Phosphorus: 47mg;

Potassium: 56mg; Sodium: 18mg

159.   Easy Flavored Potatoes Mix

Preparation time: 10 minutes

Cooking time: 25 minutes

Servings: 2

Ingredients:

- 4 potatoes, thinly sliced

- 2 tablespoons olive oil

- 1 fennel bulb, thinly sliced

- 1 tablespoon dill, chopped

- 8 cherry tomatoes, halved

- Salt and black pepper to the taste

Directions:

1. Turn on your air fryer to 365 degrees f and add the oil.

2. Add potato slices, fennel, dill, tomatoes, salt and pepper, toss, cover and cook for 25 minutes.

3. Divide potato mix between plates and serve.

4. Enjoy!

Nutrition:

Calories 240, Fat 3, Fiber 2,

Carbs 5, Protein 12

160.   Vegetarian Summer Rolls

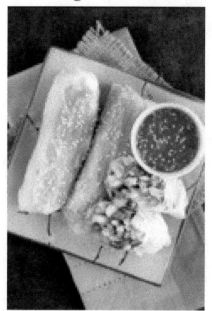

Preparation Time: 3. Minutes

Cooking Time: 0 minute

Servings: 24

Ingredients:

- 1 ounce of rice vermicelli noodles

- 2 zucchinis shredded

- 2 carrots shredded

- 2 shallots finely chopped

- 2 small cucumbers peeled and diced

- 1/3 cup of fresh basil chopped

- ½ cup of fresh cilantro chopped

- 24 spring roll wrappers

Dipping Sauce:

- 1/4 cup of sugar

- 1/4 cup of rice vinegar

- 2 fresh red chilies

Directions:

1. Place sugar, vinegar, and 2 tbsp. of water in a saucepan and boil gently.

2. Remove from heat, add chilies, and set aside.

3. In a large bowl, combine all rest of the ingredients (except wrappers).

4. Place a moistened wrapper on a work surface.

5. Put a spoonful of filling in the center and fold to encase, bringing corner to corner.

6. Fold in sides and roll up tightly. Brush end with water to seal.

7. Repeat until all filling is used.

8. Serve with dipping sauce.

Nutrition:

Calories: 94.5

Protein: 0.2g

Sodium: 562.6mg

Phosphorus: 0.5mg

Potassium: 34.0mg

161. Roasted Red Pepper Hummus

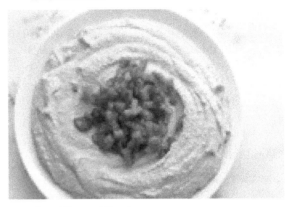

Preparation Time: 10 minutes

Cooking Time: 10 minutes

Servings: 8

Ingredients:

- 1 red bell pepper

- 1 (15-ounce) can of chickpeas, drained and rinsed

- Juice of 1 lemon

- 2 tablespoons of tahini

- 2 garlic cloves

- 2 tablespoons of extra-virgin olive oil

Directions:

1. Move the rack of the oven to the highest position. Heat the broiler to high.

2. Core the pepper and cut it into three or four large pieces. Arrange them on a baking sheet, skin-side up.

3. Broil the peppers for 5 to 10 minutes, until the skins are charred. Remove from the oven then transfer the peppers to a small bowl. Cover with plastic wrap and let them steam for 10 to 15 minutes, until cool enough to handle.

4. Peel the charred skin off the peppers, and place the peppers in a blender.

5. Add the chickpeas, lemon juice, tahini, garlic, and olive oil. Wait until smooth, then add up to 1 tablespoon of water to adjust consistency as desired.

Nutrition:

Calories: 103

Total Fat: 6g

Saturated Fat: 1g

Cholesterol: 0mg

Carbohydrates: 10g

Fiber: 3g

Protein: 3g

Phosphorus: 58mg

Potassium: 91mg

Sodium: 72mg

162. Thai-Style Eggplant Dip

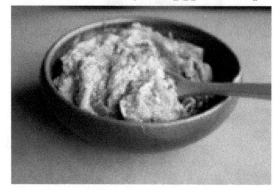

Preparation Time: 10 minutes

Cooking Time: 30 minutes

Servings: 4

Ingredients:

- 1 pound of Thai eggplant (or Japanese or Chinese eggplant)

- 2 tablespoons of rice vinegar

- 2 teaspoons of sugar

- 1 teaspoon of low-sodium soy sauce

- 1 jalapeño pepper

- 2 garlic cloves

- ¼ cup of chopped basil

- Cut vegetables or crackers, for serving

Directions:

1. Preheat the oven to 425°F to get it ready.

2. Pierce every eggplant with a skewer or knife. Place on a rimmed baking sheet and cook until soft, about 30 minutes. Let cool, cut in half, and scoop out the flesh of the eggplant into a blender.

3. Add the rice vinegar, sugar, soy sauce, jalapeño, garlic, and basil to the blender. Process until smooth. Serve with cut vegetables or crackers.

Nutrition:

Calories: 40 Total Fat: 0g Saturated Fat: 0g

Cholesterol: 0mg Carbohydrates: 10g

Fiber: 4g Protein: 2g Phosphorus: 34mg

Potassium: 284mg Sodium: 47mg

163. Coconut Pancakes

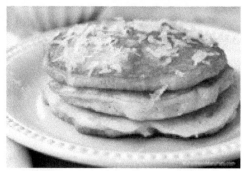

Preparation Time: 5 minutes

Cooking Time: 10 minutes

Servings: 2

Ingredients:

- 2 free-range egg whites

- 2 tbsp. of all-purpose white flour

- 3 tbsp. of coconut shavings
- 2 tbsp. of coconut milk (optional)
- 1 tbsp. of coconut oil

Directions:

1. Get a bowl and combine all the ingredients.

2. Mix well until you get a thick batter.

3. Heat a skillet on medium heat and heat the coconut oil.

4. Pour half the mixture to the center of the pan, forming a pancake and cook through for 3-4 minutes on each side.

5. Serve with your choice of berries on the top.

Nutrition:

Calories: 177 Fat: 13g

Carbohydrates: 12g Phosphorus: 37mg

Potassium: 133mg Sodium: 133mg

Protein: 5g

164.   Spiced Peaches

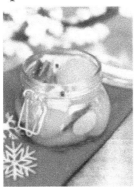

Preparation Time: 5 minutes

Cooking Time: 10 minutes

Servings: 2

Ingredients:

- 1 cup of canned peaches in their juices
- 1/2 tsp. of cornstarch

- 1 tsp. of ground cloves
- 1 tsp. of ground cinnamon
- 1 tsp. of ground nutmeg
- 1/2 lemon zest
- 1/2 cup of water

Directions:

1. Drain peaches.

2. Combine water, cornstarch, cinnamon, nutmeg, ground cloves, and lemon zest in a pan on the stove.

3. Heat on medium heat and add peaches.

4. Bring to a boil, reduce the heat and simmer for 10 minutes.

5. Serve warm.

Nutrition:

Calories: 70 Fat: 1g Carbohydrates: 18g

Phosphorus: 26mg Potassium: 184mg

Sodium: 9mg Protein: 1g

165.   Pumpkin Cheesecake Bar

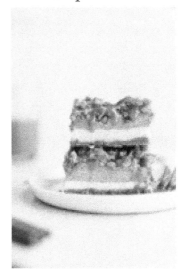

Preparation Time: 10 minutes

Cooking Time: 50 minutes

Servings: 4

Ingredients:

- 2 ½ tbsp. of unsalted butter

- 4 oz. of cream cheese
- 1/2 cup of all-purpose white flour
- 3 tbsp. of golden brown sugar
- 1/4 cup of granulated sugar
- 1/2 cup of puréed pumpkin
- 2 egg whites
- 1 tsp. of ground cinnamon
- 1 tsp. of ground nutmeg
- 1 tsp. of vanilla extract

Directions:

1. Set the oven 350 degree F/170 degree C/Gas Mark 4 for Preheating.
2. Mix the flour and brown sugar in a mixing bowl.
3. Mix in the butter with your fingertips to form 'breadcrumbs.'
4. Place 3/4 of this mixture into the bottom of an ovenproof dish.
5. Bake in the oven for 15 minutes and remove to cool.
6. Lightly whisk the egg and fold in the cream cheese, sugar (or substitute stevia), pumpkin, cinnamon, nutmeg, and vanilla until smooth.
7. Pour this mixture over the oven-baked base and sprinkle with the rest of the breadcrumbs from earlier.
8. Place back in the oven and bake for a further 30–35 minutes.
9. Allow to cool and slice to serve.

Nutrition:

Calories: 296

Fat: 17g

Carbohydrates: 30g

Phosphorus: 62mg

Potassium: 164g

Sodium: 159mg

Protein: 5g

166. Blueberry and Vanilla Mini Muffins

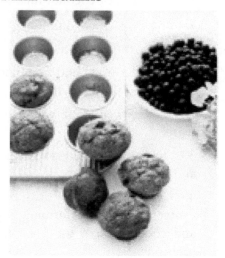

Preparation Time: 10 minutes

Cooking Time: 35 minutes

Servings: 5

Ingredients:

- 3 egg whites
- 1/4 cup of all-purpose white flour
- 1 tbsp. of coconut flour
- 1 tsp. of baking soda
- 1 tbsp. of nutmeg, grated
- 1 tsp. of vanilla extract
- 1 tsp. of stevia
- 1/4 cup of fresh blueberries

Directions:

1. Set the oven 325°F/170°C/Gas Mark 3 for Preheating.
2. Add all the ingredients in a bowl.
3. Divide the batter into 4 and spoon into a lightly oiled muffin tin.
4. Bake in the oven for 15–20 minutes or until cooked through.
5. Your knife should pull out clean from the middle of the muffin once done.

6. Allow to cool on a wired rack before serving.

Nutrition:

Calories: 48

Fat: 1g

Carbohydrates: 8g

Phosphorus: 14mg

Potassium: 44mg

Sodium: 298mg

Protein: 2g

167. Puffy French Toast

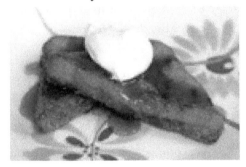

Preparation Time: 10 minutes

Cooking Time: 8 minutes

Servings: 4

Ingredients:

- 4 slices of white bread, cut in half diagonally
- 3 whole eggs and 1 egg white
- 1 cup of plain almond milk
- 2 tbsp. of canola oil
- 1 tsp. of cinnamon

Directions:

1. Preheat your oven to 400F/180C

2. Beat the eggs and the almond milk.

3. Heat the oil in a pan.

4. Dip each bread slice/triangle into the egg and almond milk mixture.

5. Fry in the pan until golden brown on each side.

6. Place the toasts in a baking sheet and let cook in the oven for another 5 minutes.

7. Serve warm and drizzle with some honey, icing sugar, or cinnamon on top.

Nutrition:

Calories: 293.75

Carbohydrate: 25.3g

Protein: 9.27g

Sodium: 211g

Potassium: 97mg

Phosphorus: 165mg

Dietary Fiber: 12.3g

Fat: 16.50g

168. Puff Oven Pancakes

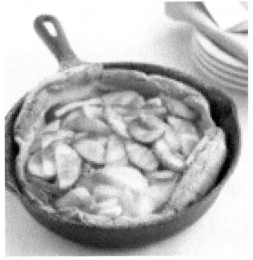

Preparation Time: 5 minutes

Cooking Time: 30 minutes

Servings: 4

Ingredients:

- 2 large eggs.
- ½ cup of rice flour
- ½ cup of rice milk

- 2 tbsp. of unsalted butter
- 1/8 tsp. of salt

Directions:

1. Preheat the oven at 400°F/190°C.

2. Grease a 10-inch skillet or Pyrex with the butter and heat in the oven until it melts.

3. Beat the eggs and whisk in the rice milk, flour and salt in a mixing bowl until smooth.

4. Take off the skillet or pie dish from the oven.

5. Transfer the batter directly into the skillet and put back in the oven for 25–30 minutes.

6. Place in a serving dish and cut into 4 portions.

7. Serve hot with honey or icing sugar on top.

Nutrition:

Calories: 159.75 Carbohydrate: 17g

Protein: 5g Sodium: 120g Potassium: 52mg

Phosphorus: 66.25mg Dietary Fiber: 0.5g

Fat: 9g

169. Savory Muffins with Protein

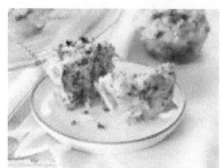

Preparation Time: 5 minutes

Cooking Time: 35 minutes

Servings: 12

Ingredients:

- 2 cups of corn flakes
- ½ cup of unfortified almond milk
- 4 large eggs
- 2 tbsp. of olive oil
- 1/2 cup of almond milk
- 1 medium white onion, sliced
- 1 cup of plain Greek yogurt
- ¼ cup of pecans, chopped
- 1 tbsp. of mixed seasoning blend, e.g., Mrs. dash

Directions:

1. Preheat the oven at 350°F/180°C.

2. Heat the olive oil in the pan. Saute the onions with the pecans and seasoning blend for a couple of minutes.

3. Add the rest of the ingredients and toss well.

4. Split the mixture into 12 small muffin cups (lightly greased) and bake for 30–35 minutes or until an inserted knife or toothpick is coming out clean.

5. Serve warm or keep at room temperature for a couple of days.

Nutrition:

Calories: 106.58

Carbohydrate: 8.20g

Protein: 4.77g

Sodium: 51.91mg

Potassium: 87.83 mg

Phosphorus: 49.41 mg

Dietary Fiber: 0.58 g

Fat: 5 g

CHAPTER 8:

Breakfast Recipes for Those who have Dialysis

170.   Cottage Cheese Pancakes

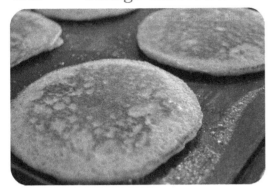

Preparation time: 5 minutes

Cooking Time: 10 minutes

Servings: 4

Ingredients:

- 1 cup cottage cheese
- 1/3 cup all-purpose flour
- 2 tablespoons vegetable oil
- 3 eggs, lightly beaten

Direction:

1. Begin by beating the eggs in a suitable bowl then stir in the cottage cheese.
2. Once it is well mixed, stir in the flour.
3. Pour a teaspoon of vegetable oil in a non-stick griddle and heat it.
4. Add 1/4 cup of the batter in the griddle and cook for 2 minutes per side until brown.
5. Cook more of the pancakes using the remaining batter.

Nutrition:

Calories 196

Total Fat 11.3g

Saturated Fat 3.1g

Cholesterol 127mg

Sodium 276mg

Protein 13g

Calcium 58mg

Phosphorous 187 mg

Potassium 110mg

171.   Asparagus Bacon Hash

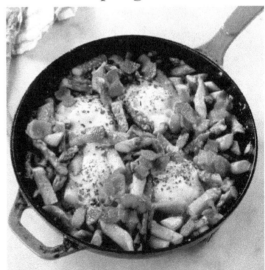

Preparation time: 5 minutes

Cooking Time: 27 minutes

Servings: 4

Ingredients:

- 6 slices bacon, diced
- 1/2 onion, chopped

- 2 cloves garlic, sliced

- 2 lb. asparagus, trimmed and chopped

- Black pepper, to taste

- 2 tablespoons Parmesan, grated

- 4 large eggs

- 1/4 teaspoon red pepper flakes

Direction:

1. Add the asparagus and a tablespoon of water to a microwave proof bowl.

2. Cover the veggies and microwave them for 5 minutes until tender.

3. Set a suitable non-stick skillet over moderate heat and layer it with cooking spray.

4. Stir in the onion and sauté for 7 minutes, then toss in the garlic.

5. Stir for 1 minute, then toss in the asparagus, eggs, and red pepper flakes.

6. Reduce the heat to low and cover the vegetables in the pan. Top the eggs with Parmesan cheese.

7. Cook for approximately 15 minutes, then slice to serve.

Nutrition:

Calories 290

Total Fat 17.9g

Saturated Fat 6.1g

Cholesterol 220mg

Sodium 256mg

Protein 23.2g

Calcium 121mg

Phosphorous 247mg

Potassium 715mg

172.   Cheese Spaghetti Frittata

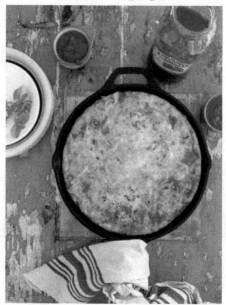

Preparation time: 5 minutes

Cooking Time: 10 minutes

Servings: 6

Ingredients:

- 4 cups whole-wheat spaghetti, cooked

- 4 teaspoons olive oil

- 3 medium onions, chopped

- 4 large eggs

- ½ cup milk

- 1/3 cup Parmesan cheese, grated

- 2 tablespoons fresh parsley, chopped

- 2 tablespoons fresh basil, chopped

- ½ teaspoon black pepper

- 1 tomato, diced

Direction:

1. Set a suitable non-stick skillet over moderate heat and add in the olive oil.

2. Place the spaghetti in the skillet and cook by stirring for 2 minutes on moderate heat.

3. Whisk the eggs with milk, parsley, and black pepper in a bowl.

4. Pour this milky egg mixture over the spaghetti and top it all with basil, cheese, and tomato.

5. Cover the spaghetti frittata again with a lid and cook for approximately 8 minutes on low heat.

6. Slice and serve.

Nutrition:

Calories 230 Total Fat 7.8g Saturated Fat 2g

Cholesterol 127mg Sodium 77mg

Protein 11.1g Calcium 88mg

Phosphorous 368 mg

Potassium 214mg

173.   Pineapple Bread

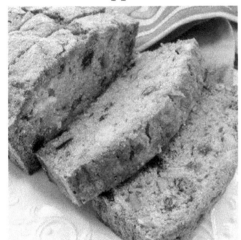

Preparation time: 5 minutes

Cooking Time: 1 hour

Servings: 10

Ingredients:

- 1/3 cup Swerve
- 1/3 cup butter, unsalted
- 2 eggs
- 2 cups flour
- 3 teaspoons baking powder
- 1 cup pineapple, undrained
- 6 cherries, chopped

Direction:

1. Whisk the Swerve with the butter in a mixer until fluffy.

2. Stir in the eggs, then beat again.

3. Add the baking powder and flour, then mix well until smooth.

4. Fold in the cherries and pineapple.

5. Spread this cherry-pineapple batter in a 9x5 inch baking pan.

6. Bake the pineapple batter for 1 hour at 350 degrees F.

7. Slice the bread and serve.

Nutrition:

Calories 197 Total Fat 7.2g

Saturated Fat 1.3g Cholesterol 33mg

Sodium 85mg Protein 4g

Calcium 79mg Phosphorous 316mg

Potassium 227mg

174.   Parmesan   Zucchini Frittata

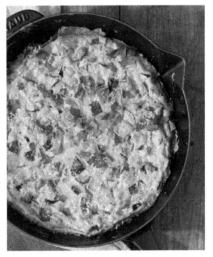

Preparation time: 5 minutes

Cooking Time: 35 minutes

Servings: 6

Ingredients:

- 1 tablespoon olive oil
- 1 cup yellow onion, sliced

- 3 cups zucchini, chopped
- ½ cup Parmesan cheese, grated
- 8 large eggs
- ½ teaspoon black pepper
- 1/8 teaspoon paprika
- 3 tablespoons parsley, chopped

Direction:

1. Toss the zucchinis with the onion, parsley, and all other ingredients in a large bowl.
2. Pour this zucchini-garlic mixture in an 11x7 inches pan and spread it evenly.
3. Bake the zucchini casserole for approximately 35 minutes at 350 degrees F.
4. Cut in slices and serve.

Nutrition:

Calories 142 Total Fat 9.7g

Saturated Fat 2.8g Cholesterol 250mg

Sodium 123mg Protein 10.2g

Calcium 73mg Phosphorous 375mg

Potassium 286mg

175.   Texas Toast Casserole

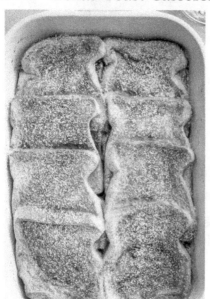

Preparation time: 10 minutes

Cooking Time: 30 minutes

Servings: 10

Ingredients:

- 1/2 cup butter, melted
- 1 cup brown Swerve
- 1 lb. Texas Toast bread, sliced
- 4 large eggs
- 1 1/2 cup milk
- 1 tablespoon vanilla extract
- 2 tablespoons Swerve
- 2 teaspoons cinnamon
- Maple syrup for serving

Direction:

1. Layer a 9x13 inches baking pan with cooking spray.
2. Spread the bread slices at the bottom of the prepared pan.
3. Whisk the eggs with the remaining ingredients in a mixer.
4. Pour this mixture over the bread slices evenly.
5. Bake the bread for 30 minutes at 350 degrees F in a preheated oven.

Nutrition:

Calories 332

Total Fat 13.7g

Saturated Fat 6.9g

Cholesterol 102mg

Sodium 350mg

Protein 7.4g

Calcium 143mg

Phosphorous 186mg

Potassium 74mg

176. Apple Cinnamon Rings

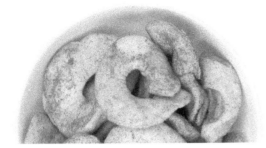

Preparation time: 10 minutes

Cooking Time: 20 minutes

Servings: 6

Ingredients:

- 4 large apples, cut in rings
- 1 cup flour
- 1/4 teaspoon baking powder
- 1 teaspoon stevia
- 1/4 teaspoon cinnamon
- 1 large egg, beaten
- 1 cup milk
- Vegetable oil, for frying
- Cinnamon Topping:
- 1/3 cup of brown Swerve
- 2 teaspoons cinnamon

Direction:

1. Begin by mixing the flour with the baking powder, cinnamon, and stevia in a bowl.
2. Whisk the egg with the milk in a bowl.
3. Stir in the dry flour mixture and mix well until it makes a smooth batter.
4. Pour oil into a wok to deep fry the rings and heat it up to 375 degrees F.
5. First, dip the apple in the flour batter and deep fry until golden brown.
6. Transfer the apple rings on a tray lined with paper towel.
7. Drizzle the cinnamon and Swerve topping over the slices.
8. Serve fresh in the morning.

Nutrition:

Calories 166

Total Fat 1.7g

Saturated Fat 0.5g

Cholesterol 33mg

Sodium 55mg

Protein 4.7g

Calcium 65mg

Phosphorous 241mg

Potassium 197mg

177. Zucchini Bread

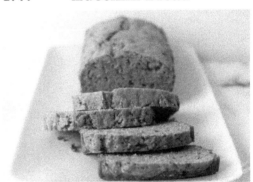

Preparation time: 10 minutes

Cooking Time: 1 hour

Servings: 16

Ingredients:

- 3 eggs
- 1 1/2 cups Swerve
- 1 cup apple sauce
- 2 cups zucchini, shredded
- 1 teaspoon vanilla
- 2 cups flour
- 1/4 teaspoon baking powder
- 1 teaspoon baking soda

- 1 teaspoon cinnamon
- 1/2 teaspoon ginger
- 1 cup unsalted nuts, chopped

Direction:

1. Thoroughly whisk the eggs with the zucchini, apple sauce, and the rest of the ingredients in a bowl.
2. Once mixed evenly, spread the mixture in a loaf pan.
3. Bake it for 1 hour at 375 degrees F in a preheated oven.
4. Slice and serve.

Nutrition:

Calories 200

Total Fat 5.4g

Saturated Fat 0.9g

Cholesterol 31mg

Sodium 94mg

Protein 4.4g

Calcium 20mg

Phosphorous 212mg

Potassium 137mg

178.   Garlic Mayo Bread

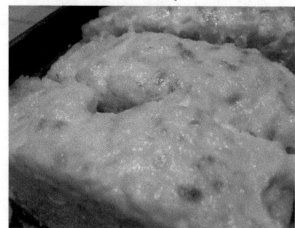

Preparation time: 5 minutes

Cooking Time: 5 minutes

Servings: 16

Ingredients:

- 3 tablespoons vegetable oil
- 4 cloves garlic, minced
- 2 teaspoons paprika
- Dash cayenne pepper
- 1 teaspoon lemon juice
- 2 tablespoons Parmesan cheese, grated
- 3/4 cup mayonnaise
- 1 loaf (1 lb.) French bread, sliced
- 1 teaspoon Italian herbs

Direction:

1. Mix the garlic with the oil in a small bowl and leave it overnight.
2. Discard the garlic from the bowl and keep the garlic-infused oil.
3. Mix the garlic-oil with cayenne, paprika, lemon juice, mayonnaise, and Parmesan.
4. Place the bread slices in a baking tray lined with parchment paper.
5. Top these slices with the mayonnaise mixture and drizzle the Italian herbs on top.
6. Broil these slices for 5 minutes until golden brown.
7. Serve warm.

Nutrition:

Calories 217

Total Fat 7.9g

Saturated Fat 1.8g

Cholesterol 5mg

Sodium 423mg

Protein 7g

Calcium 56mg

Phosphorous 347mg

Potassium 72mg

179. Strawberry Topped Waffles

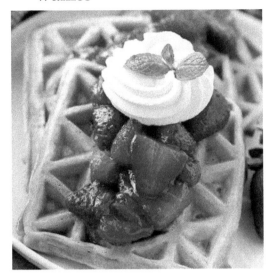

Preparation time: 5 minutes

Cooking Time: 20 minutes

Servings: 5

Ingredients:

- 1 cup flour
- 1/4 cup Swerve
- 1 3/4 teaspoons baking powder
- 1 egg, separated
- 3/4 cup milk
- ½ cup butter, melted
- ½ teaspoon vanilla extract
- Fresh strawberries, sliced

Direction:

1. Prepare and preheat your waffle pan following the Direction of the machine.
2. Begin by mixing the flour with Swerve and baking soda in a bowl.
3. Separate the egg yolks from the egg whites, keeping them in two separate bowls.
4. Add the milk and vanilla extract to the egg yolks.
5. Stir the melted butter and mix well until smooth.
6. Now beat the egg whites with an electric beater until foamy and fluffy.
7. Fold this fluffy composition in the egg yolk mixture.
8. Mix it gently until smooth, then add in the flour mixture.
9. Stir again to make a smooth mixture.
10. Pour a half cup of the waffle batter in a preheated pan and cook until the waffle is done.
11. Cook more waffles with the remaining batter.
12. Serve fresh with strawberries on top.

Nutrition:

Calories 342

Total Fat 20.5g

Saturated Fat 12.5g

Cholesterol 88mg

Sodium 156mg

Protein 4.8g

Calcium 107mg

Phosphorous 126mg

Potassium 233mg

CHAPTER 9:

Lunch Recipes for the Those who have Dialysis

180.   Chicken Noodle Soup

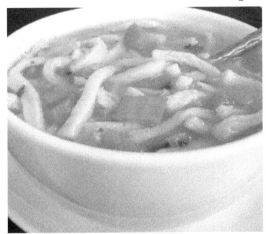

Preparation Time: 15 minutes

Cooking Time: 25 minutes

Servings: 4

Ingredients:

- 1 cup low-sodium chicken broth
- 1 cup water
- 1/4 teaspoon poultry seasoning
- 1/4 teaspoon black pepper
- 1/4 cup carrot, chopped
- 1 cup chicken, cooked and shredded
- 2 ounces egg noodles

Direction:

1. Add broth and water in a slow cooker.
2. Set the pot to high.
3. Add poultry seasoning and pepper.
4. Add carrot, chicken and egg noodles to the pot.

5. Cook on high setting for 25 minutes.
6. Serve while warm.

Nutrition:

Calories 141 Protein 15 g

Carbohydrates 11 g Fat 4 g

Cholesterol 49 mg Sodium 191 mg

Potassium 135 mg Phosphorus 104 mg

Calcium 16 mg Fiber 0.7 g

181.   Beef Stew with Apple Cider

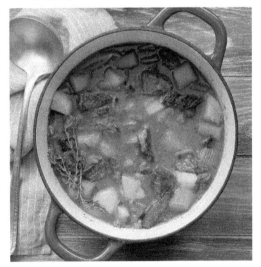

Preparation Time: 15 minutes

Cooking Time: 10 hours

Servings: 8

Ingredients:

- 1/2 cup potatoes, cubed
- 2 lb. beef cubes
- 7 tablespoons all-purpose flour, divided

- 1/4 teaspoon thyme
- Black pepper to taste
- 3 tablespoons oil
- ¼ cup carrot, sliced
- 1 cup onion, diced
- 1/2 cup celery, diced
- 1 cup apples, diced
- 2 cups apple cider
- 1/2 cups water
- 2 tablespoons apple cider vinegar

Direction:

1. Double boil the potatoes (to reduce the amount of potassium) in a pot of water.
2. In a shallow dish, mix the half of the flour, thyme and pepper.
3. Coat all sides of beef cubes with the mixture.
4. In a pan over medium heat, add the oil and cook the beef cubes until brown. Set aside.
5. Layer the ingredients in your slow cooker.
6. Put the carrots, potatoes, onions, celery, beef and apple.
7. In a bowl, mix the cider, vinegar and 1 cup water.
8. Add this to the slow cooker.
9. Cook on low setting for 10 hours.
10. Stir in the remaining flour to thicken the soup.

Nutrition:

Calories 365 Protein 33 g

Carbohydrates 20 g Fat 17 g

Cholesterol 73 mg Sodium 80 mg

Potassium 540 mg Phosphorus 234 mg

Calcium 36 mg Fiber 2.2 g

182.   Chicken Chili

Preparation Time: 20 minutes

Cooking Time: 1 hour and 15 minutes

Servings: 8

Ingredients:

- 1 tablespoon oil
- 1 cup onion, chopped
- 4 garlic cloves, chopped
- 1 cup green pepper
- 1 cup celery, chopped
- 1 cup carrots, chopped
- 14 oz. low-sodium chicken broth
- 1 lb. chicken breast, cubed and cooked
- 1 cup low-sodium tomatoes, drained and iced
- 1 cup kidney beans, rinsed and drained
-                     3/4 cup salsa
- 3 tablespoons chili powder
- 1 teaspoon ground oregano
- 4 cups white rice, cooked

Direction:

1. In a pot, pour oil and cook onion, garlic, green pepper, celery and carrots.
2. Add the broth.
3. Bring to a boil.
4. Add the rest of the ingredients except the rice.
5. Simmer for 1 hour.
6. Serve with rice.

Nutrition:

Calories 355 Protein 24 g

Carbohydrates 38 gFat 12 g

Cholesterol 59 mg Sodium 348 mg

Potassium 653 mg Phosphorus 270 mg

Calcium 133 mg Fiber 4.7 g

Lamb Stew

Preparation Time: 30 minutes

Cooking Time: 1 hour and 40 minutes

Servings: 6

Ingredients:

- 1 lb. boneless lamb shoulder, trimmed and cubes
- Black pepper to taste
- 1/4 cup all-purpose flour
- 1 tablespoon olive oil
- 1 onion, chopped
- 3 garlic cloves, chopped
- 1/2 cup tomato sauce
- 2 cups low-sodium beef broth
- 1 teaspoon dried thyme
- 2 parsnips, sliced
- 2 carrots, sliced
- 1 cup frozen peas

Direction:

1. Season lamb with pepper.
2. Coat evenly with flour.
3. Pour oil in a pot over medium heat.
4. Cook the lamb and then set aside.
5. Add onion to the pot.
6. Cook for 2 minutes.
7. Add garlic and saute for 30 seconds.
8. Pour in the broth to deglaze the pot.
9. Add the tomato sauce and thyme.
10. Put the lamb back to the pot.
11. Bring to a boil and then simmer for 1 hour.
12. Add parsnips and carrots.
13. Cook for 30 minutes.
14. Add green peas and cook for 5 minutes.

Nutrition:

Calories 283

Protein 27 g

Carbohydrates 19 g

Fat 11 g

Cholesterol 80 mg

Sodium 325 mg

Potassium 527 mg

Phosphorus 300 mg

Calcium 56 mg

Fiber 3.4 g

183.   Tofu Stir Fry

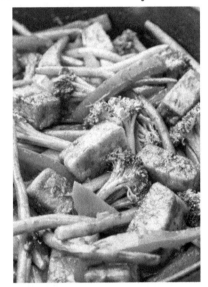

Preparation Time: 15 minutes

Cooking Time: 20 minutes

Servings: 4

Ingredients:

- 1 teaspoon sugar
- 1 tablespoon lime juice
- 1 tablespoon low sodium soy sauce
- 2 tablespoons cornstarch
- 2 egg whites, beaten
- ½ cup unseasoned bread crumbs
- 1 tablespoon vegetable oil

- 16 ounces tofu, cubed
- 1 clove garlic, minced
- 1 tablespoon sesame oil
- 1 red bell pepper, sliced into strips
- 1 cup broccoli florets
- 1 teaspoon herb seasoning blend
- Dash black pepper
- Sesame seeds
- Steamed white rice

Direction:

1. Dissolve sugar in a mixture of lime juice and soy sauce. Set aside.
2. In the first bowl, put the cornstarch.
3. Add the egg whites in the second bowl.
4. Place the breadcrumbs in the third bowl.
5. Dip each tofu cubes in the first, second and third bowls.
6. Pour vegetable oil in a pan over medium heat.
7. Cook tofu cubes until golden.
8. Drain the tofu and set aside.
9. Remove oil from the pan and add sesame oil.
10. Add garlic, bell pepper and broccoli.
11. Cook until crisp tender
12. Season with the seasoning blend and pepper.
13. Put the tofu back and toss to mix.
14. Pour soy sauce mixture on top and transfer to serving bowls.
15. Garnish with the sesame seeds and serve on top of white rice.

Nutrition:

Calories 400

Protein 19 g

Carbohydrates 45 g

Fat 16 g

Cholesterol 0 mg

Sodium 584 mg

Potassium 317 mg

Phosphorus 177 mg

Calcium 253 mg

Fiber 2.7 g

184.   Broccoli Pancake

Preparation Time: 10 minutes

Cooking Time: 5 minutes

Servings: 4

Ingredients:

- 3 cups broccoli florets, diced
- 2 eggs, beaten
- 2 tablespoons all-purpose flour
- 1/2 cup onion, chopped
- 2 tablespoons olive oil

Direction:

1. Boil broccoli in water for 5 minutes. Drain and set aside.
2. Mix egg and flour.
3. Add onion and broccoli to the mixture.
4. Pour oil in a pan over medium heat.
5. Cook the broccoli pancake until brown on both sides.

Nutrition:

Calories 140

Protein 6 g

Carbohydrates 7 g

Fat 10 g

Cholesterol 106 mg

Sodium 58 mg

Potassium 276 mg

Fiber 2.1 g

185.   Carrot Casserole

Preparation Time: 10 minutes

Cooking Time: 20 minutes

Serving: 8

Ingredients:

- 1 lb. carrots, sliced into rounds
- 12 low-sodium crackers
- 2 tablespoons butter
- 2 tablespoons onion, chopped
- 1/4 cup cheddar cheese, shredded

Direction:

1. Preheat your oven to 350 degrees F.
2. Boil carrots in a pot of water until tender.
3. Drain the carrots and reserve ¼ cup liquid.
4. Mash carrots.
5. Add all the ingredients into the carrots except cheese.
6. Place the mashed carrots in a casserole dish.
7. Sprinkle cheese on top and bake in the oven for 15 minutes.

Nutrition:

Calories 94

Protein 2 g

Carbohydrates 9 g

Fat 6 g

Cholesterol 13 mg

Sodium 174 mg

Potassium 153 mg

Phosphorus 47 mg

Calcium 66 mg

Fiber 1.8 g

186.   Cauliflower Rice

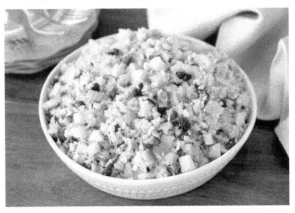

Preparation Time: 10 minutes

Cooking Time: 10 minutes

Servings: 4

Ingredients:

- 1 head cauliflower, sliced into florets
- 1 tablespoon butter
- Black pepper to taste
- 1/4 teaspoon garlic powder
- 1/4 teaspoon herb seasoning blend

Direction:

1. Put cauliflower florets in a food processor.
2. Pulse until consistency is similar to grain.
3. In a pan over medium heat, melt the butter and add the spices.
4. Toss cauliflower rice and cook for 10 minutes.
5. Fluff using a fork before serving.

Nutrition:

Calories 47 Protein 1 g

Carbohydrates 4 g Fat 3 g

Cholesterol 8 mg Sodium 43 mg

Potassium 206 mg

Phosphorus 31 mg

Calcium 16 mg

187.   Chicken Pineapple Curry

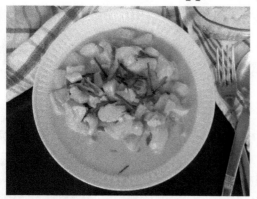

Preparation Time: 10 minutes

Cooking Time: 3 hours 10 minutes

Servings: 6

Ingredients:

- 1 1/2 lbs. chicken thighs, boneless, skinless
- 1/2 teaspoon black pepper
- 1/2 teaspoon garlic powder
- 2 tablespoons olive oil
- 20 oz. canned pineapple
- 2 tablespoons brown Swerve
- 2 tablespoons soy sauce
- 1/2 teaspoon Tabasco sauce
- 2 tablespoons cornstarch
- 3 tablespoons water

Direction:

1. Begin by seasoning the chicken thighs with garlic powder and black pepper.
2. Set a suitable skillet over medium-high heat and add the oil to heat.
3. Add the boneless chicken to the skillet and cook for 3 minutes per side.
4. Transfer this seared chicken to a Slow cooker, greased with cooking spray.

5. Add 1 cup of the pineapple juice, Swerve, 1 cup of pineapple, tabasco sauce, and soy sauce to a slow cooker.
6. Cover the chicken-pineapple mixture and cook for 3 hours on low heat.
7. Transfer the chicken to the serving plates.
8. Mix the cornstarch with water in a small bowl and pour it into the pineapple curry.
9. Stir and cook this sauce for 2 minutes on high heat until it thickens.
10. Pour this sauce over the chicken and garnish with green onions.
11. Serve warm.

Nutrition:

Calories 256 Total Fat 10.4g

Saturated Fat 2.2g Cholesterol 67mg

Sodium 371mg Total Carbohydrate 13.6g

Dietary Fiber 1.5g Sugars 8.4g

Protein 22.8g Calcium 28mg

Phosphorous 107 mg Potassium 308mg

188.   Baked Pork Chops

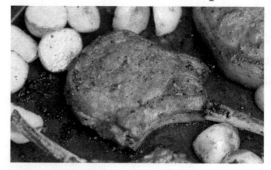

Preparation Time: 10 minutes

Cooking Time: 40 minutes

Servings: 6

Ingredients:

- 1/2 cup flour

- 1 large egg

- 1/4 cup water

- 3/4 cup breadcrumbs

- 6 (3 1/2 oz.) pork chops

- 2 tablespoons butter, unsalted

- 1 teaspoon paprika

Direction:

1. Begin by switching the oven to 350 degrees F to preheat.

2. Mix and spread the flour in a shallow plate.

3. Whisk the egg with water in another shallow bowl.

4. Spread the breadcrumbs on a separate plate.

5. Firstly, coat the pork with flour, then dip in the egg mix and then in the crumbs.

6. Grease a baking sheet and place the chops in it.

7. Drizzle the pepper on top and bake for 40 minutes.

8. Serve.

Nutrition:

Calories 221

Total Fat 7.8g

Saturated Fat 1.9g

Cholesterol 93mg

Sodium 135mg

Protein 24.7g

Calcium 13mg

Phosphorous 299mg

Potassium 391mg

CHAPTER 10:

Dinner Recipes for those who Have Dialysis

189. Lemon Pepper Trout

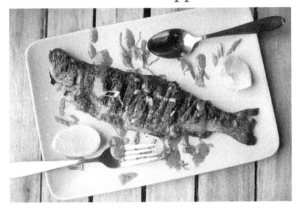

Preparation Time: 5 minutes

Cooking Time: 15 minutes

Servings: 2

Ingredients:

- 1 lb. trout fillets
- 1 lb. asparagus
- 3 tablespoons olive oil
- 5 garlic cloves, minced
- 1/2 teaspoon black pepper
- 1/2 lemon, sliced

Direction:

1. Prepare and preheat the gas oven at 350 degrees F.
2. Rub the washed and dried fillets with oil then place them in a baking tray.
3. Top the fish with lemon slices, black pepper, and garlic cloves.
4. Spread the asparagus around the fish.

5. Bake the fish for 15 minutes approximately in the preheated oven.
6. Serve warm.

Nutrition:

Calories 336 Total Fat 20.3g

Saturated Fat 3.2g

Cholesterol 84mg

Sodium 370mg

Protein 33g

Calcium 100mg

Phosphorous 107mg

Potassium 383mg

190. Salmon Stuffed Pasta

Preparation Time: 10 minutes

Cooking Time: 35 minutes

Servings: 24

Ingredients:

- 24 jumbo pasta shells, boiled
- 1 cup coffee creamer

Filling:

- 2 eggs, beaten
- 2 cups creamed cottage cheese
- ¼ cup chopped onion
- 1 red bell pepper, diced
- 2 teaspoons dried parsley
- ½ teaspoon lemon peel
- 1 can salmon, drained

Dill Sauce:

- 1 1/2 teaspoon butter
- 1 1/2 teaspoon flour
- 1/8 teaspoon pepper
- 1 tablespoon lemon juice
- 1 ½ cup coffee creamer
- 2 teaspoons dried dill weed

Direction:

1. Beat the egg with the cream cheese and all the other filling ingredients in a bowl.
2. Divide the filling in the pasta shells and place the bodies in a 9x13 baking dish.
3. Pour the coffee creamer around the stuffed shells then cover with a foil.
4. Bake the shells for 30 minutes at 350 degrees F.
5. Meanwhile, whisk all the ingredients for dill sauce in a saucepan.
6. Stir for 5 minutes until it thickens.
7. Pour this sauce over the baked pasta shells.
8. Serve warm.

Nutrition:

Calories 268

Total Fat 4.8g

Saturated Fat 2g

Cholesterol 27mg

Sodium 86mg

Protein 11.5g

Calcium 27mg

Phosphorous 314mg

Potassium 181mg

191.   Tuna Casserole

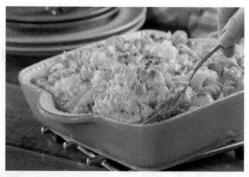

Preparation Time: 15 minutes

Cooking time: 35 minutes

Servings: 4

Ingredients:

- ½ cup Cheddar cheese, shredded
- 2 tomatoes, chopped
- 7 oz tuna filet, chopped
- 1 teaspoon ground coriander
- ½ teaspoon salt
- 1 teaspoon olive oil
- ½ teaspoon dried oregano

Directions:

1. Brush the casserole mold with olive oil.
2. Mix up together chopped tuna fillet with dried oregano and ground coriander.
3. Place the fish in the mold and flatten well to get the layer.
4. Then add chopped tomatoes and shredded cheese.
5. Cover the casserole with foil and secure the edges.
6. Bake the meal for 35 minutes at 355F.

Nutrition:

Calories 260, Fat 21.5, Fiber 0.8, Carbs 2.7,

Protein 14.6Sodium 80mg Calcium 58mg

Phosphorous 220mg Potassium 241mg

192. Oregano Salmon with Crunchy Crust

Preparation Time: 10 minutes

Cooking time: 2 hours

Servings: 2

Ingredients:

- 8 oz salmon fillet
- 2 tablespoons panko bread crumbs
- 1 oz Parmesan, grated
- 1 teaspoon dried oregano
- 1 teaspoon sunflower oil

Directions:

1. In the mixing bowl combine panko bread crumbs, Parmesan, and dried oregano.
2. Sprinkle the salmon with olive oil and coat in the breadcrumbs mixture.
3. After this, line the baking tray with baking paper.
4. Place the salmon in the tray and transfer in the preheated to the 385F oven.
5. Bake the salmon for 25 minutes.

Nutrition:

Calories 245,

Fat 12.8,

Fiber 0.6,

Carbs 5.9,

Protein 27.5

Sodium 80mg

Calcium 78mg

Phosphorous 230mg

Potassium 331mg

193. Sardine Fish Cakes

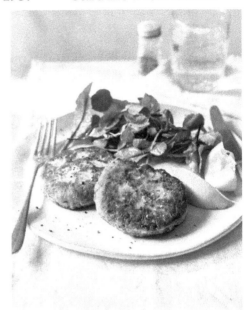

Preparation Time: 10 minutes

Cooking time: 10 minutes

Servings: 4

Ingredients:

- 11 oz sardines, canned, drained
- 1/3 cup shallot, chopped
- 1 teaspoon chili flakes
- ½ teaspoon salt
- 2 tablespoon wheat flour, whole grain
- 1 egg, beaten
- 1 tablespoon chives, chopped
- 1 teaspoon olive oil
- 1 teaspoon butter

Directions:

1. Put the butter in the skillet and melt it.
2. Add shallot and cook it until translucent.
3. After this, transfer the shallot in the mixing bowl.
4. Add sardines, chili flakes, salt, flour, egg, chives, and mix up until smooth with the help of the fork.

5. Make the medium size cakes and place them in the skillet.

6. Add olive oil.

7. Roast the fish cakes for 3 minutes from each side over the medium heat.

8. Dry the cooked fish cakes with the paper towel if needed and transfer in the serving plates.

Nutrition:

Calories 221,

Fat 12.2,

Fiber 0.1,

Carbs 5.4,

Protein 21.3

Sodium 80mg

Calcium 98mg

Phosphorous 230mg

Potassium 241mg

194.   Cajun Catfish

Preparation Time: 10 minutes

Cooking time: 10 minutes

Servings: 4

Ingredients:

- 16 oz catfish steaks (4 oz each fish steak)
- 1 tablespoon cajun spices
- 1 egg, beaten
- 1 tablespoon sunflower oil

Directions:

1. Pour sunflower oil in the skillet and preheat it until shimmering.

2. Meanwhile, dip every catfish steak in the beaten egg and coat in Cajun spices.

3. Place the fish steaks in the hot oil and roast them for 4 minutes from each side.

4. The cooked catfish steaks should have a light brown crust.

Nutrition:

Calories 263, Fat 16.7, Fiber 0,

Carbs 0.1, Protein 26.3

Sodium 60mg

Calcium 78mg

Phosphorous 250mg

Potassium 231mg

195.   Teriyaki Tuna

Preparation Time: 10 minutes

Cooking time: 6 minutes

Servings: 3

Ingredients:

- 3 tuna fillets
- 3 teaspoons teriyaki sauce
- ½ teaspoon minced garlic
- 1 teaspoon olive oil

Directions:

1. Whisk together teriyaki sauce, minced garlic, and olive oil.

2. Brush every tuna fillet with teriyaki mixture.

3. Preheat grill to 390F.

4. Grill the fish for 3 minutes from each side.

Nutrition:

Calories 382,

Fat 32.6,

Fiber 0,

Carbs 1.1,

Protein 21.4

Sodium 80mg

Calcium 78mg

Phosphorous 230mg

Potassium 331mg

196. Herbed Vegetable Trout

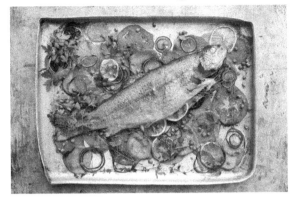

Preparation Time: 10 minutes

Cooking Time: 15 minutes

Servings: 4

Ingredients:

- 14 oz. trout fillets
- 1/2 teaspoon herb seasoning blend
- 1 lemon, sliced
- 2 green onions, sliced
- 1 stalk celery, chopped
- 1 medium carrot, julienne

Direction:

1. Prepare and preheat a charcoal grill over moderate heat.
2. Place the trout fillets over a large piece of foil and drizzle herb seasoning on top.
3. Spread the lemon slices, carrots, celery, and green onions over the fish.
4. Cover the fish with foil and pack it.
5. Place the packed fish in the grill and cook for 15 minutes.
6. Once done, remove the foil from the fish.
7. Serve.

Nutrition:

Calories 202

Total Fat 8.5g

Saturated Fat 1.5g

Cholesterol 73mg

Sodium 82mg

Protein 26.9g

Calcium 70mg

Phosphorous 287mg

Potassium 560mg

197. Citrus Glazed Salmon

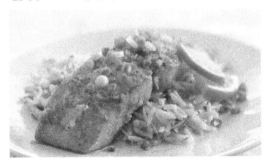

Preparation Time: 10 minutes

Cooking Time: 17 minutes

Servings: 4

Ingredients:

- 2 garlic cloves, crushed
- 1 1/2 tablespoons lemon juice
- 2 tablespoons olive oil
- 1 tablespoon butter
- 1 tablespoon Dijon mustard
- 2 dashes cayenne pepper
- 1 teaspoon dried basil leaves
- 1 teaspoon dried dill
- 24 oz. salmon filet

Direction:

1. Place a 1-quart saucepan over moderate heat and add the oil, butter, garlic, lemon juice, mustard, cayenne pepper, dill, and basil to the pan.
2. Stir this mixture for 5 minutes after it has boiled.

3. Prepare and preheat a charcoal grill over moderate heat.

4. Place the fish on a foil sheet and fold the edges to make a foil tray.

5. Pour the prepared sauce over the fish.

6. Place the fish in the foil in the preheated grill and cook for 12 minutes.

7. Slice and serve.

Nutrition:

Calories 401

Total Fat 20.5g

Saturated Fat 5.3g

Cholesterol 144mg

Sodium 256mg

Protein 48.4g

Calcium 549mg

Phosphorous 214mg

Potassium 446mg

198. Broiled Salmon Fillets

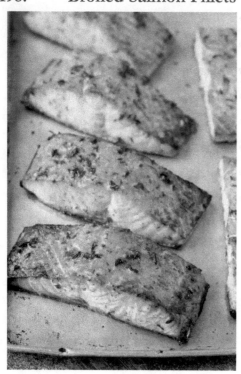

Preparation Time: 10 minutes

Cooking Time: 13 minutes

Servings: 4

Ingredients:

- 1 tablespoon ginger root, grated
- 1 clove garlic, minced
- ¼ cup maple syrup
- 1 tablespoon hot pepper sauce
- 4 salmon fillets, skinless

Direction:

1. Grease a pan with cooking spray and place it over moderate heat.

2. Add the ginger and garlic and sauté for 3 minutes then transfer to a bowl.

3. Add the hot pepper sauce and maple syrup to the ginger-garlic.

4. Mix well and keep this mixture aside.

5. Place the salmon fillet in a suitable baking tray, greased with cooking oil.

6. Brush the maple sauce over the fillets liberally

7. Broil them for 10 minutes at the oven at broiler settings.

8.   Serve warm.

Nutrition:

Calories 289

Total Fat 11.1g

Saturated Fat 1.6g

Cholesterol 78mg

Sodium 80mg

Protein 34.6g

Calcium 78mg

Phosphorous 230mg

Potassium 331mg

CHAPTER 11:

21 Days Meal Plan

Day	Breakfast	Lunch	Dinner
1	Garlic Mayo Bread	Salad with Vinaigrette	Beef Soup
2	Strawberry Topped Waffles	Salad with Lemon Dressing	Amazing Grilled Chicken and Blueberry Salad
3	Cheese Spaghetti Frittata	Shrimp with Salsa	Clean Chicken and Mushroom Stew
4	Shrimp Bruschetta	Cauliflower Soup	Elegant Pumpkin Chili Dish
5	Strawberry Muesli	Cabbage Stew	Zucchini Zoodles with Chicken and Basil
6	Yogurt Bulgur	Baked Haddock	Tasty Roasted Broccoli
7	Bacon and Cheese Crustless Quiche	Herbed Chicken	The Almond Breaded Chicken Goodness
8	Mushroom Crustless Quiche	Pesto Pork Chops	South-Western Pork Chops
9	Maple Glazed Walnuts	Vegetable Curry	Almond butter Pork Chops
10	Ham and Cheese Strata	Grilled Steak with Salsa	Chicken Salsa
11	Breakfast Salad from Grains and Fruits	Buffalo Chicken Lettuce Wraps	Healthy Mediterranean Lamb Chops
12	French toast with Applesauce	Crazy Japanese Potato and Beef Croquettes	Amazing Sesame Breadsticks
13	Bagels Made Healthy	Saucy Garlic Greens	Brown Butter Duck Breast
14	Cornbread with Southern Twist	Garden Salad	Generous Garlic Bread Stick
15	Grandma's Pancake Special	Spicy Cabbage Dish	Cauliflower Bread Stick

16		Very Berry Smoothie	Extreme Balsamic Chicken	Bacon and Chicken Garlic Wrap
17		Pasta with Indian Lentils	Enjoyable Spinach and Bean Medley	Chipotle Lettuce Chicken
18		Pineapple Bread	Tantalizing Cauliflower and Dill Mash	Eggplant and Red Pepper Soup
19		Parmesan Zucchini Frittata	Secret Asian Green Beans	Seafood Casserole
20		Texas Toast Casserole	Excellent Acorn Mix	Ground Beef and Rice Soup
21		Cornbread with Southern Twist	Sporty Baby Carrots	Couscous Burgers

Conclusion

Y ou likely had little knowledge about your kidneys before. You probably didn't know how you could take steps to improve your kidney health and decrease the risk of developing kidney failure. However, through reading this book, you now understand the power of the human kidney, as well as the prognosis of chronic kidney disease. While over thirty-million Americans are being affected by kidney disease, you can now take steps to be one of the people who is actively working to promote your kidney health. Kidney disease now ranks as the 18th deadliest condition in the world. In the United States alone, it is reported that over 600,000 Americans succumb to kidney failure.

These stats are alarming, which is why, it is necessary to take proper care of your kidneys, starting with a kidney-friendly diet. These recipes are ideal whether you have been diagnosed with a kidney problem or you want to prevent any kidney issue.

With regards to your wellbeing and health, it's a smart thought to see your doctor as frequently as conceivable to ensure you don't run into preventable issues that you needn't get. The kidneys are your body's toxin channel (just like the liver), cleaning the blood of remote substances and toxins that are discharged from things like preservatives in food & other toxins. At the point when you eat flippantly and fill your body with toxins, either from nourishment, drinks (liquor or alcohol for instance) or even from the air you inhale (free radicals are in the sun and move through your skin, through messy air, and numerous food sources contain them). Your body additionally will in general convert numerous things that appear to be benign until your body's organs convert them into things like formaldehyde because of a synthetic response and transforming phase.

One case of this is a large portion of those diet sugars utilized in diet soft drinks for instance, Aspartame transforms into Formaldehyde in the body. These toxins must be expelled, or they can prompt ailment, renal (kidney) failure, malignant growth, & various other painful problems.

This isn't a condition that occurs without any forethought it is a dynamic issue and in that it very well may be both found early and treated, diet changed, and settling what is causing the issue is conceivable. It's conceivable to have partial renal failure yet, as a rule; it requires some time (or downright awful diet for a short time) to arrive at absolute renal failure. You would prefer not to reach total renal failure since this will require standard dialysis treatments to save your life.

Dialysis treatments explicitly clean the blood of waste and toxins in the blood utilizing a machine in light of the fact that your body can no longer carry out the responsibility. Without treatments, you could die a very painful death. Renal failure can be the consequence of long-haul diabetes, hypertension, unreliable diet, and can stem from other health concerns.

A renal diet is tied in with directing the intake of protein and phosphorus in your eating routine. Restricting your sodium intake is likewise significant. By controlling these two variables you can control the vast majority of the toxins/waste made by your body and thus this enables your kidney to 100% function. In the event that you get this early enough and truly moderate your diets with extraordinary consideration, you could avert all-out renal failure. In the event that you get this early, you can take out the issue completely.